MIDWIFERY PRACTICE

Intrapartum Care

A research-based approach

Edited by

Jo Alexander, Valerie Levy
and *Sarah Roch*

MACMILLAN

First published 1990 by
THE MACMILLAN PRESS LTD
Houndmills, Basingstoke, Hampshire RG21 2XS
and London
Companies and representatives
throughout the world

ISBN 0–333–53862–5 hardcover
ISBN 0–333–51370–3 paperback

A catalogue record for this book is available
from the British Library.

Reprinted 1991 (twice), 1992, 1993, 1994

Printed in Malaysia

Contents

Other volumes in the Midwifery Practice series

■ **Antenatal Care**   ISBN 0–333–51369–X (paperback)
                         ISBN 0–333–53861–7 (hardcover)

1. *Joyce Shorney*: Preconception care: the embryo of health promotion
2. *Rosemary Currell*: The organisation of midwifery care
3. *Rosemary C. Methven*: The antenatal booking interview
4. *Jo Alexander*: Antenatal preparation of the breasts for breastfeeding
5. *Moira Plant*: Maternal alcohol and tobacco use during pregnancy
6. *Tricia Murphy-Black*: Antenatal education
7. *Jean Proud*: Ultrasound: the midwife's role
8. *Joyce Prince and Margaret Adams*: The psychology of pregnancy
9. *Jane Spillman*: Multiple births – parents' anxieties and the realities

■ **Postnatal care**   ISBN 0–333–51371–1 (paperback)
                        ISBN 0–333–53863–3 (hardcover)

1. *Jennifer Sleep*: Postnatal perineal care
2. *Sally Inch*: Postnatal care relating to breastfeeding
3. *Jenifer M. Holden*: Emotional problems associated with childbirth
4. *Ellena Salariya*: Parental-infant attachment
5. *Janet Rush*: Care of the umbilical cord
6. *Chris Whitby*: Transitional care
7. *Margaret Adams and Joyce Prince*: Care of the grieving parent, with special reference to stillbirth
8. *Rowan Nunnerley*: Quality assurance in postnatal care
9. *Marianne J. G. Mills*: Teenage mothers

Contributors to this volume

Janette Brierley RGN RM ADM MTD PGCEA
School of Midwifery, St Mary's Hospital, London.
Janette Brierley, a midwife teacher, won a scholarship in 1986 which enabled a visit to New York to observe midwifery practice in a high HIV-prevalence area. This lead to an increasing involvement with HIV antibody positive women. While remaining clinically very active, she speaks at many major conferences and is on the management committee of Positively Women.

Rona Campbell BSc MSc PhD
University of Ulster at Jordanstown.
While a doctoral student, Rona Campbell completed a national survey of home births and, together with medical statistician Alison Macfarlane, has undertaken an extensive review of the evidence and debate on place of birth. She is now a lecturer in social research methods.

Sheila Drayton RGN RM MTD MSc
Nursing Officer, Welsh Office, Cardiff.
Sheila Drayton has practised as a midwife and nurse in the UK and in Malawi. Her former post as Director of Midwifery allowed her to combine her research interests, including clinical practice in midwifery and client satisfaction, with the development of midwifery care wards, offering continuity of care to women. She is a member of the Welsh National Board.

Judith Grant BEdHons MTD RM RGN
Worcester and District School of Midwifery.
Judith Grant qualified as a midwife from Queen Mothers' Hospital Glasgow and as a midwife teacher from Surrey University. She has taught midwifery in Hastings and Cornwall prior to becoming senior tutor in Worcester. She is at present studying for an MEd degree.

Christine Henderson MA SRN SCM DipN(Lond) MTD
Birmingham & Solihull College of Midwifery.
Apart from undertaking research relating to rupture of the membranes,

vi · *Contributors to this volume*

Christine Henderson has helped a group of midwives to develop a framework for midwifery practice. She is interested in the professional development of midwives and in teaching in clinical practice, and is about to conduct a research study evaluating the ENB 997 course. She is vice-principal and head of midwifery and related studies, with a special responsibility for continuing education.

Alison M Heywood BSc RGN RM Diploma in Social Research
Chase Farm Hospital, Enfield, Middlesex.
Having worked in a variety of maternity units in Southern England, Alison Heywood is currently a senior midwife/team leader. Previous research posts include studies of TENS, provision of epidural services, and community antenatal clinics.

Elaine Ho RGN RM ADM MTD PGCEA MSc in Social Research BA
Dorset and Salisbury College of Midwifery and Nursing.
Elaine Ho is head of midwifery education with a main interest in the carrying out of sociological research in the midwifery field.

Valerie Levy MPhil RM RGN MTD
Southwest College of Health Studies/University of Plymouth.
Valerie Levy is a Series Editor and details about her are given on the back cover of this book.

Carolyn Roth BA SRN SCM MTD PGCEA
Department of Community Health and Nursing Studies, Southbank Polytechnic, London.
Carolyn Roth has been a midwife teacher since 1983. Her interest in HIV in pregnancy is part of a more general concern to help promote a practice of midwifery which places women and their varied needs at the centre of decisions about care.

Jennifer Sleep SRN SCM MTD BA
Royal Berkshire Hospital, Reading.
Jennifer Sleep is co-ordinator of nursing and midwifery research within the West Berkshire Health Authority. She has conducted a series of clinical trials designed to evaluate aspects of midwifery care largely related to perineal management both during delivery and following childbirth.

Foreword

I am pleased and privileged to be able to welcome this important and timely book. At a time when midwives and students are clamouring for sound information about good research which relates to their day-to-day practice, this book provides an excellent resource.

Until recently, midwives who wanted to know more about their practice had two options. They could use textbooks which were based mainly on clinical experience (important, but of limited use in helping to decide between fact and opinion), or they could tackle the huge and often inaccessible range of research literature in journals (also important, but time-consuming and often hard to relate to day-to-day practice).

The editors and authors of this volume and its two companion volumes provide us with a third option. They have aimed to bring together the best of published research with the best of clinical wisdom. To this end, authors who are experts in their own clinical fields describe and interpret the evidence, and give clear guidelines (not rules) for practice. We are approaching a time when we will no longer be able to carry out a practice 'because we have always done it this way', or 'because I was told to do it'. We will be expected to give care based on sound information: this volume provides us with some of that information.

You can use this book in different ways. It can be used as a text for teaching senior students, or for midwives to bring themselves up to date with recent developments. Or it could be used as a first step into a more in-depth study of the literature: the extensive reference lists will be very valuable.

The most encouraging aspect of this book for me is the lack of didactic rules. Instead, the very varied wishes and needs of the women and families we care for are put first by every author. Our care should be based on awareness of those needs and wishes, then it should be shaped by the information arising from existing research evidence. The result is an adult approach to midwifery, where we take the best of all worlds: caring, science and experience.

This book makes a great contribution to that adult approach. I welcome its publication, and I congratulate the editors and authors on their skill and vision.

Mary J Renfrew
Bsc RGN SCM PhD
Oxford, June 1990

Preface

There is no doubt that the theory underpinning midwifery practice cannot be carved in tablets of stone but must be dynamic and change as new information becomes available. Despite this, it is really only in the last 30 years that research has begun to have any impact on midwifery practice and even now relevant information is not always easily available to practitioners. The Midwives Information and Resource Service (MIDIRS) and the 'Research and the Midwife' conferences have made an outstanding contribution, but standard textbooks are often sparsely referenced and full length research papers are time consuming to read.

This three volume series is intended to help to fill the vacuum which exists between the current state of research and the literature readily available and accessible to practitioners. The series offers midwives and senior student midwives a broad-ranging survey and analysis of the research literature relating to the major areas of clinical practice. We hope that it will also prove stimulating to childbearing women, their families and others involved with the maternity care services. The books do not pretend to give the comprehensive coverage of a definitive textbook and indeed their strength derives from the in-depth treatment of a selection of topics. The topic areas were chosen with great care and authors were approached who have a particular research interest and expertise. On the basis of their critical appraisal of the literature the authors make recommendations for clinical practice, and thus the predominant feature of these books is the link made between research and key areas of practice.

The chapters have a common structure which is described below. It is hoped that this will be attractive to readers and assist those reviewing existing policies or wishing to study a topic in still greater depth. Some knowledge of basic research terminology will prove useful, but its lack should not discourage readers.

We owe a debt of gratitude to many people: most of all to our authors who have worked so painstakingly to produce their contributions and many of whom have helped us in numerous other ways; to Sarah Robinson for her early encouragement and to our publishers during the development of the series; and, not least, to all those practitioners and students who made valuable comments on draft material.

We hope that many practitioners will use the books to increase their knowledge, stimulate their interest in research and improve and extend their own practice of the art and science of midwifery.

JA
VL
SR

■ Common structure of chapters

In fulfilment of the aims of the series, each chapter follows a common structure:

1. The introduction offers a digest of the contents;

2. *'It is assumed that you are already aware of the following . . .'* establishes the prerequisite knowledge and experience assumed of the reader;

3. The main body of the chapter reviews and analyses the most appropriate and important research literature currently available;

4. The *'Recommendations for clinical practice'* offer suggestions for sound clinical practice based on the author's interpretation of the literature;

5. The *'Practice check'* enables professionals to examine their own practice and the principles and policies influencing their work;

6. Bibliographic sources are covered under *References* (to research) and *Suggestions for further reading.*

■ Further reading on research

The titles listed below are suggested for those who wish to further their knowledge and understanding of research principles.

Cormack D F S (ed) 1984 The Research Process in Nursing. Blackwell Scientific Publications, Oxford

Hockey L 1985 Nursing Research – Mistakes and Misconceptions. Churchill Livingstone, Edinburgh

Tornquist E M 1986 From proposal to publication: an informal guide to writing about nursing research. Addison Wesley, Reading (Massachusetts)

Chapter 1

The place of birth

Rona Campbell

> It is clearly unsatisfactory to base the provision of maternity beds solely on obstetric needs; preferences, home conditions, and domestic ties must be taken into account. The maternity services cater in the main for healthy women going through a normal physiological process; their needs, therefore, are more complex than those of the sick, where the clinical aspect is all-important.
>
> (Joint Committee of the RCOG and the Population Investigation Committee 1948)

> As unforseen complications can occur in any birth, every mother should be encouraged to have her baby in a maternity unit where emergency facilities are readily available.
>
> (Maternity Services Advisory Committee 1984)

These statements, both made by committees set up to investigate and make recommendations on the maternity services and separated by a period of 36 years, help to illustrate the enormous change that has taken place in the way in which childbirth is viewed. In the first quotation childbirth is viewed as a 'normal' process experienced by 'healthy women'. The second statement on the other hand portrays a view of childbirth as a pathological process in which medical intervention may well be required.

This change in perspective has occurred at the same time as other important developments in maternity care; notably the move from delivery at home to delivery in hospital and the increasing use of technology in the 'management' of labour and delivery.

This chapter aims to look at some of the reasons why this change in thinking occurred and the implications this has had for policy on place of birth. In particular the chapter will focus on the role that scientific evidence of the relative merits and demerits of the various places of birth has played in the formulation of policy recommendations about where women should give birth.

Current policy on place of birth is based on two assumptions: firstly, that hospital is the safest place to give birth and secondly that the overall decline in perinatal mortality has been due to an increase in the percentage of births taking place in hospital. These two assumptions will be challenged and some rather different conclusions drawn.

■ It is assumed that you are already aware of the following:

- The definition of a perinatal mortality rate;
- The reasons why it is important to compare rates and proportions rather than absolute numbers;
- The differences between observational and experimental research methods;
- What the statistical term 'correlation' means and what a spurious correlation is.

■ Recent thinking on place of birth

In 1927 when the Office of the Registrar General for England and Wales first published data on the numbers of births by place of delivery, 15 per cent of live births were recorded as having taken place in institutions (Registrar General 1928). By the time the Population Investigation Committee (1948) carried out its research into maternity services in Great Britain this figure had risen to 54 per cent and, as predicted in the report, the percentage of hospital deliveries has continued to increase. By 1981 only one per cent of births took place at home. Since 1981 the proportion of births at home has remained fairly constant but the trend towards care in large consultant obstetric units has continued.

These changes have been encouraged by successive committees charged with investigating and making recommendations about the maternity services, and have been underpinned by a substantial shift in thinking about safety and the place of birth.

On the basis of an analysis of obstetric text books published between 1960 and 1980, Eckart Schwarz (1990) has argued that up until the 1960s the obstetrician's role was to deal with the abnormal and in particular with problems relating to the mechanics of labour. With the increase of births in hospital during the 1950s and 1960s, however, he suggests that the category of what was abnormal expanded and was accompanied by increased rates of intervention. This, it is suggested, led to a quite radical shift in the conception of the role and responsibilities of the obstetrician.

The traditional dichotomy of normal childbirth versus childbirth with distinct abnormalities was absorbed into the new concept of abnormality as representing a dynamic departure from normal physiological functioning.

Thus,

> Instead of being mechanics responsible for the mending of faults, they became engineers in charge of the smooth running of 'all systems' so that faults did not even occur. The obstetric engineer has to master and control normal physiology in order to prevent the abnormal from happening.
>
> (Schwarz, 1990)

This new thinking led to suggestions that a birth could only be considered normal in retrospect and, because of the potential of any birth becoming abnormal, that all births should be conducted in hospital (or in the view of some, an intensive care situation) so that labour could be carefully monitored and 'managed'. This kind of thinking has been equated with the military 'maxim' strategy that all planning should be based on the worst possible scenario (Brody & Thompson 1981).

Given this background it was not altogether surprising that in 1970 the Peel Report stated:

> We consider that the resources of modern medicine should be available to all mothers and babies, and we think that sufficient facilities should be provided to allow for 100% hospital delivery. The greater safety of hospital confinement justifies this objective.
>
> (DHSS 1970)

Judged by the small proportion of births now taking place at home the implementation of this policy appears to have been successful. The debate about where women should give birth is, however, far from over. While there has been this change in thinking amongst many involved in the provision of maternity services, others have remained sceptical and in some cases strongly opposed to the view that every birth should be treated as potentially abnormal. The debate has remained unresolved, partly because of these differing perspectives on birth and partly because the scientific effectiveness of many of the new strategies adopted in the light of this new thinking, both in terms of place of birth and the management of labour, were not tested before they were widely recommended and implemented. As the following review of the scientific evidence relating to the place of birth shows, had policy on place of birth been made on the basis of scientific evidence, a rather different pattern of maternity care might have emerged.

■ Evaluating outcomes by place of delivery

One of the most important difficulties in trying to make sense of the evidence on place of birth relates to outcome measures. The most widely used measure of pregnancy outcome is perinatal mortality. This, however, is a very crude indicator of the quality of perinatal care. The two major determinants of perinatal death are lethal congenital malformations and the pathology associated with low birthweight. Thus, before comparisons between outcomes for different places of delivery are made these factors should be taken into account (Chalmers & Macfarlane 1980). In many studies, unfortunately, this has not been done.

The quality of maternity care can also be measured in terms of morbidity and the degree of satisfaction with the service. The decline in perinatal mortality means that these indicators have become increasingly important.

A further difficulty is that the place of delivery is not synonymous with the type of care provided. Women giving birth in an NHS hospital may do so in a consultant unit, in a general practitioner (GP) bed in a consultant unit, in a GP unit which may or may not be on the same hospital site as a consultant obstetric unit, or possibly in one of the new midwifery units where women are cared for entirely by midwives. The pattern of antenatal care received can also vary as can the person actually conducting the delivery.

All of the research undertaken on place of birth has involved collection and analysis of observational rather than experimental data. The difficulty here is that with correlational rather than experimental evidence there is no certainty that differences in outcomes can actually be attributed solely to differences in the place of birth.

Perinatal deaths are now so rare and the numbers of births outside hospitals with consultant obstetric facilities so low that it would be impossible to conduct a trial that was sufficiently large to detect statistically significant differences in perinatal mortality among babies to low risk women (Lilford 1987), although experimental work is now being used to evaluate new ways of providing maternity care (Flint *et al* 1989).

■ Rates of institutional delivery and perinatal mortality

One of the most persistent features of policy on place of birth in the UK is the suggestion, expressed here by the chair of the Maternity Advisory Services Committee, Alison Munro:

> The practice of delivering nearly all babies in hospital has
> contributed to the dramatic reduction in stillbirths and neonatal
> deaths and to the avoidance of many child handicaps.
> (Maternity Services Advisory Committee 1984)

A similar assumption was made by the Peel Committee when it recommended universal hospital delivery and the same view has recently been put forward by the government in response to a parliamentary question.

> We aim to minimise the risks to babies by encouraging delivery in hospital preferably with access to the full range of facilities which are likely to be found only on district general hospital sites ... As a result there has been a fall in perinatal mortality in England from 14.6 per thousand births in 1979 to 9.8 in 1985.
>
> (Hansard 1987)

Constant repetition does not make something true and detailed analyses (see below) of the temporal association between the increase in the rate of institutional delivery and the decline in the overall rate of perinatal mortality strongly suggest that the association is coincidental.

Marjorie Tew (1978) could find no association between yearly changes in the percentage of hospital births and rates of perinatal mortality in 15 UK hospital board regions for the period 1962–71, and only a negative association for the years 1969–78. A similar study (Fryer & Ashford 1972; Ashford 1978) based on local authority areas in England and Wales for the period 1955 to 1973 showed that higher hospital delivery rates were associated with lower mortality rates for babies weighing less than 2501 grams but that the converse was true from 1964 onwards for babies above this weight. These findings also seem to be supported by more recent evidence from the Netherlands where home deliveries have always formed an important part of the maternity services. A regional study of the percentage of deliveries in hospital and perinatal mortality rates (Treffers & Laan 1986) failed to detect any association. Furthermore, the decline in perinatal mortality in Denmark (where hospital birth has been favoured) and the Netherlands has been remarkably similar in spite of very different policies towards the place of birth (Scherjon 1986).

Evidence from two local maternity surveys further calls into question the existence of a causal link. In Newcastle upon Tyne between 1960 and 1969 perinatal mortality declined uniformly among hospital and home births (Barron *et al* 1977). Data from the Cardiff births survey (Chalmers *et al* 1976) however showed that while the ratio of home to hospital births fell from one in five to one in a hundred between 1963 and 1973, there was no statistically significant improvement in perinatal mortality nor any reduction in deaths from causes deemed preventable.

Since 1980 the percentage of births occurring at home in England and Wales has remained almost static at around one per cent of all births while the overall perinatal mortality rate has fallen by 29 per cent, again suggesting that factors other than the decline in home deliveries are responsible for the reduction in perinatal mortality.

It is unfortunate that so much recent policy on place of birth seems to be based on an assumption which is not supported by any scientific evidence. Regrettably the words written by Irish playwright George Bernard Shaw in the introduction to his play 'The Doctor's Dilemma' in 1906 seem equally relevant today.

> Simple and obvious as this is, nobody seems as yet to discount the effect of substituting attention for neglect in drawing conclusions from health statistics. Everything is put to the credit of the particular method employed, although it may quite possibly be raising the death-rate by five per thousand whilst the attention incidental to it is reducing the death-rate fifteen per thousand. The net gain of ten per thousand is credited to the method, and made the excuse for enforcing more of it.

■ Perinatal mortality and place of birth

Until 1949, data on place of birth compiled by the General Register Office for England and Wales did not include perinatal mortality rates by place of birth. In this year however a special exercise was undertaken to link birth registration particulars with the death registration of any infant dying during the first year of life. Thus it would have been possible to produce perinatal mortality rates by place of delivery for this linked data set.

Such analyses were not performed on the grounds that:

> A direct comparison of the safety to mother and child in hospital delivery as opposed to domiciliary confinement, as at present organized, is vitiated because known difficult cases are normally booked for hospital and emergencies are rushed there. In fact, in any such comparison, it is usual for the death rates to be higher in hospital than at home, though no informed person would adduce this particular fact as evidence that it is more dangerous to have a baby in hospital.
>
> (Heady & Morris 1956)

This quote is interesting because it highlights two important difficulties encountered when attempting to examine perinatal outcome according to the place of birth; the first is a statistical problem, the second one of politics.

Since the inception of the Ministry of Health in 1919 the policy has always been to encourage the selective referral to hospital of all those women for whom an adverse outcome of pregnancy seemed more likely (Ministry of Health 1920). In addition, social processes have meant that women with different backgrounds may have been selected, or themselves have chosen, different places in which to give birth. Thus, place of birth analyses are confounded by selection factors which may be related both to the place of delivery and the outcome.

The political problem arises because the idea that hospital obstetric care might enhance the risk of a poor outcome for some women is such an anathema to many that attempts to address this question are likely to be resisted and findings which challenge the prevailing view dismissed whatever the merits or demerits of the statistical analysis.

One way of controlling for selection biases is to standardise perinatal mortality rates for different places of birth to take into account the different proportions of women or babies possessing characteristics associated with an increased risk of death. Early attempts at employing this technique involved standardisation for single risk factors (Senn undated; Ashford 1978; Tew 1978). This approach, although an improvement on comparisons based on crude perinatal mortality rates was nevertheless unsatisfactory because no single factor could be expected to account for all differences in mortality between birth locations.

Subsequent analyses by Marjorie Tew (1985a) were more sophisticated in that she employed two composite risk scores which incorporated a variety of risk factors. These antenatal (APS) and labour (LPS) prediction scores had been constructed by other researchers from data collected in a national survey of births in 1958 and applied to data from a similar survey undertaken in 1970.

Data indicating labour prediction scores and the attendant perinatal mortality for births classified according to the place of delivery were not published in the original report of this survey but after some protracted negotiations were eventually made available to Tew. The results of her (1985) analysis are shown in Table 1.1.

Table 1.1   Births and perinatal mortality rates (PNMRs) by labour prediction score and place of delivery

Level of risk	LPS	All births		Percentage of births at each score		PNMR per 1000	
		Number	Per cent	Hospital	GP unit & home†	Hospital	GP unit & home†
Very low	1–2	7488	45.9	58.7	41.3	8.0	3.9*
Low	2	3723	22.8	68.8	31.2	17.9	5.2**
Moderate	3	2273	13.9	76.6	23.4	32.2	3.8***
High	4–6	2417	14.8	84.0	16.0	53.2	15.5**
Very high	7–12	427	2.6	96.5	3.5	162.6	133.3

* p<0.05   ** p<0.005   *** p<0.001
† Includes GP beds in consultant units
Source: Tew 1985a

As expected, births which attracted higher risk scores were associated with increased rates of perinatal mortality. Within risk categories, however, there were substantial differences between rates for births in obstetric hospitals and those for home births or births in GP units. Except for the small number of births at the highest level of predicted risk, these differences were all statistically significant. On the basis of these findings Tew (1985a) concluded that, 'Unless some other factor can be found to explain these results from the obstetricians' own analysis of survey data, they must be interpreted as meaning that most infants do not benefit from active obstetric management and most of those already at higher risk benefit least.'

While these results lend no support to the conventional wisdom that hospital delivery is safest they do require cautious interpretation. Firstly, the LPS has never been widely used so its predictive abilities remain unknown. Secondly, perinatal deaths resulting from lethal congenital abnormalities, and stillbirths where the fetus was known to be dead prior to the onset of labour, were not excluded from this analysis. As an early critic (James 1977a) noted, 'Tew's implication that hospital fatalities are due to the treatment, rather than to the selection of cases is seen to be silly when one considers that a proportion of hospital stillbirths occur in women who have been admitted for the very reason that the foetus is already dead'.

Finally, subtle selection biases may not have been controlled for by this approach. Other epidemiological research has been unable to explain even half of the differences in mortality in terms of known risk factors.

Marjorie Tew has attempted to counter these last two criticisms. She suggests that intrauterine deaths and lethal congenital malformations 'make little difference to the hospitals' excess PNMR, as official data on congenital malformations show, while in the 1970 survey the mortality rate for live births in hospital was by itself more than twice the mortality rate for all births, live and still, in GP units and home' (Tew 1985b). These points are rather misleading. Not all intrauterine deaths will be due to lethal congenital malformations and not all babies dying from lethal malformations will be stillborn. Thus, the initial criticism that hospital deliveries in the 1970 survey were likely to include a disproportionate number of perinatal deaths where the outcome would not have been affected by intrapartum care remains valid.

Tew (1985b) has also argued that unidentified risk factors not included in the Labour Prediction Score could not have influenced selection policy. As this score was constructed from data collected in 1958, however, it is quite possible that factors not identified then were influencing selection twelve years later.

■ Home birth

Evidence from a variety of surveys shows that, before the mid 1970s, perinatal mortality among babies born at home was significantly lower than for babies born in consultant obstetric units. For example, in the 1970 British Births Survey the perinatal mortality rate for singleton deliveries for home births was 4.3 per 1000 births compared with a rate of 27.8 for births in consultant obstetric units (Chamberlain *et al* 1975).

The linking of birth and death registration, undertaken on an experimental basis in 1949, has been done on a routine basis by the Office of Population Censuses and Surveys since 1975. Unlike her predecessors however, Macdonald Davies (1980) the researcher presenting the first analysis of this new 'linked file', did not flinch from producing analyses of perinatal mortality by place of birth. Even so a warning was given that 'rates for place of confinement (for example, in hospital or at home) cannot easily be interpreted'. Surprisingly, given that previous *ad hoc* surveys had always shown perinatal mortality rates for births at home to be much lower than those for births occurring in hospital, these analyses showed that the perinatal mortality rate for births at home was rising and had reached a level beyond that for deliveries in hospitals with consultant obstetric facilities.

Failing to heed the warning issued, the Social Services Committee (HC 1980), who had been investigating perinatal and neonatal mortality, reproduced these findings in a report and recommended that, 'An increasing number of mothers be delivered in large units; selection of patients is improved for small consultant units and isolated GP units; and that home delivery is phased out further.'

The committee's interpretation was criticised (Tew 1981; Campbell *et al* 1982) by those who thought that the rise in perinatal mortality for births at home probably resulted from the substantial decline in the absolute number of home births, most of which would have been planned, and a consequent rise in the proportion of unplanned births. A survey (Campbell *et al* 1984) of all births occurring at home in England and Wales in 1979 confirmed this theory. Less than two thirds of births occurring at home in that year had been planned as such. The perinatal mortality for these was shown to be very low, at 4.1 per 1000 births, while the rate for births planned to occur in hospital was significantly higher at 67.5 per 1000 births.

■ Intended place of delivery

The home births survey (Campbell *et al* 1984) highlighted the importance of the intended place of delivery. Clearly, births planned to occur in hospital may actually take place at home due to premature or precipitate labour. Equally, women whose births were booked for home delivery may be transferred to hospital either during pregnancy or after the onset of labour. Thus, the perinatal mortality rate for planned home deliveries of 4.1 per 1000 births does not represent the true risk of perinatal death for home delivery in 1979. It does not take account of those mothers who had planned to give birth at home but because of the identification of a problem during pregnancy or labour transferred and gave birth in hospital. There is considerable evidence (Rees 1961; Rutter 1964; Hudson 1968; Woodall 1968; James 1977b) to show that the mortality rates associated with transfer are high, particularly when it occurs after the onset of labour. Nevertheless, it was estimated (Campbell *et al* 1984) that even if transfers in labour were taken into account in 1979, this would have only resulted in a doubling of the rate for planned home births to 8.2 per 1000 which was still well below the overall rate for births in that year of 14.6 per 1000.

As the majority of transfers are due to the emergence of a serious problem thought to require specialist supervision, the high perinatal mortality associated with these births is not unexpected. Tew (1986) has, however, advanced a different interpretation claiming that the elevated rates are caused by the interventionist obstetrics practised in hospitals, which increase the risk of an adverse outcome. Although Tew has produced reanalyses of several studies to support her case, detailed scrutiny of these and other data suggest that her argument is not supported by the available evidence (Campbell & Macfarlane 1987).

■ Morbidity and the place of birth

As perinatal mortality continues to decline increasing emphasis has been placed on the assessment of perinatal morbidity as a measure of perinatal outcome. In a number of surveys, levels of morbidity for hospital and home births have been compared. One of the earliest (Alment *et al* 1967) showed that when preterm babies and those with jaundice were excluded, rates of infection during the first 28 days of life were lower in babies born at home. Morbidity was also found to be higher in those women who gave birth in hospital. Forty-six per cent of them had either an episiotomy or a perineal tear compared with 31 per cent of those who gave birth at home.

The 1970 British Births survey showed that babies born at home were more likely to have jaundice and suffer minor infections than those born in hospital. In contrast, those born in hospital had more serious problems such as respiratory conditions, cerebral signs and fits (Chamberlain *et al* 1975). In a study of 1692 low risk women who gave birth in a variety of settings in Groningen Municipality in the Netherlands (Damstra-Wijmenga 1984), lower rates of morbidity were recorded for home births among both women and their babies. Other studies of home births (Campbell *et al* 1984; Murphy *et al* 1984) have also shown rates of morbidity to be very low among planned births.

A study (Lievaart & de Jong 1982) of the outcome of 112 normal first pregnancies in Eindhoven in the Netherlands produced rather different findings. In this study early morbidity was measured by pH, PCO_2 and base deficit in arterial cord blood and late morbidity by testing the function of the babies' central nervous system using a standard test. Comparison was made between 27 women delivered by a gynaecologist and 85 women delivered by midwives. Both early and late mortality was greater in the group delivered by midwives in which 10 neurologically non-optimal infants were identified. There were no non-optimal infants detected in the group delivered by the gynaecologist. While the influence of place of birth was ruled out, the researchers questioned midwives' ability to select and deliver only those women with normal pregnancies. Caution is required when interpreting these findings however as measurement of both early and late mortality was not undertaken blind so the possibility of observer bias cannot be ruled out.

Unfortunately, all of the morbidity studies reviewed thus far have been purely descriptive; little or no attempt has been made in them to control for selection biases. In several studies efforts have been made to reduce the effects of selection thus increasing the likelihood that observed differences in morbidity are due to differences in the place of delivery or type of care received.

A study undertaken in the United States (Mehl 1978) matched 1046 women who planned to give birth at home with a similar group of women intending to deliver in hospital. Matching was done on the basis of age, social class and obstetric risk factors. The incidence of episiotomy was nine times higher among those delivered in hospital and the incidence of second, third and fourth degree tears was also significantly higher in this group. While there were no differences in mortality or neurological impairment between the two groups, a significantly higher proportion of the babies born in hospital had neonatal complications, including birth injuries, respiratory distress lasting more than 12 hours and neonatal infections.

A retrospective study of data collected prospectively in Oxford in 1978 (Klein *et al* 1980) sought to compare the outcomes for two groups of low risk women; one group was booked for a system of shared care with delivery booked for the consultant unit and the other group was booked to be cared for by GPs and midwives only and delivered in an integrated GP unit. The use of epidural anaesthesia and pethidine was found to be considerably higher among those booked for shared care. The proportion of babies requiring intubation and with low Apgar score was found to be smaller among those delivered in the GP unit. The authors were unable to identify precisely what aspects of consultant care were responsible for the differences observed but suggested (Klein *et al* 1983) that the use of analgesia and anaesthesia required further research. A follow up study (Klein *et al* 1985), undertaken prospectively in 1981 and based on smaller numbers failed to detect such pronounced differences.

A small prospective study (Shearer 1985) of 202 women booked for home delivery and a similar group of 185 booked for consultant care in Essex between 1979 and 1985 produced similar results to those of Klein and colleagues. The induction rate for consultant booked births was double that for births booked for home delivery. A higher proportion of babies with low Apgar scores were born to women booked for consultant care and this group also experienced higher rates of episiotomy and second degree tears.

■ Where do women want to give birth?

The earliest attempt at answering this question was made by the Joint Committee of the Royal College of Obstetricians and Gynaecologists and the Population Investigation Committee (1948). In the Committee's survey of 'Social and economic aspects of childbirth', 90.5 per cent (15 130 women) of all those who gave birth in March 1946 were successfully interviewed. A whole section of the questionnaire was devoted to the 'place of confinement'.

Although considerable regional variations were observed, when women were asked the reasons for their choice of place of confinement 50.5 per cent of those who gave birth at home said they had done so because it was their preferred location. Only 16.6 per cent of those who gave birth in hospital had apparently done so because it was their preferred location. The most common reason given by women for delivering in hospital was that their home conditions were unsuitable. The authors of the survey report concluded that, 'The general indication . . . is that many women would prefer a good domiciliary maternity service, provided that some domestic help was available and housing conditions were improved.'

Subsequent national birth surveys undertaken in 1958 (Butler & Alberman 1969) and 1970 (Chamberlain *et al* 1975; Chamberlain *et al* 1978) were based only on medical information about the birth and did not involve interviews with the mother, so regrettably this is one of the very few truly comprehensive studies of the issue. Later surveys investigating women's views on the place of birth have tended to be small scale and of opportunistic, rather than random, samples of women.

Nearly all of the studies in which it has been possible to investigate the preferences of women who have experienced both home and hospital deliveries were undertaken in the 1960s and early 1970s when home births were more common. Without exception, these studies (Gordon & Elias Jones 1960; Alment *et al* 1967; Goldthorpe & Richman 1974) revealed that the vast majority of women preferred giving birth at home. A more representative postal survey (O'Brien 1978) of 2400 women who gave birth in England and Wales in 1975 found that 92 per cent of those who had a home birth but who had previously given birth in hospital, preferred home delivery. Of those who had given birth in hospital but had previously had a home delivery, only 23 per cent preferred the hospital delivery.

A similar but more recent survey of women living in Nottingham

Health District (Caplan & Madeley 1985) found that 90 per cent of those who gave birth at home would prefer home for their next delivery and a similar 88 per cent of those who delivered in hospital said they would choose hospital again next time. It was noted, however, that there was a considerable non-response to this question 'for reasons which remain obscure' according to the authors. One of these reasons might have been that because choice of place of birth is now so restricted it may seem rather irrelevant to be asked where you would like to give birth when the overwhelming majority of births take place in hospital. The reasons most often given for preferring home delivery are that it avoids separation from the rest of the family. The major reasons recorded for wanting to give birth in hospital are because women feel safer and get more rest (Joint Committee of the RCOG & Population Investigation Committee 1948; Gordon & Elias Jones 1960; Kitzinger & Davis 1978; Campbell 1979; Caplan & Madeley 1985).

As with all place of birth studies based on observational data, surveys of women's preferences are probably subject to selection biases. Women who have had an unsatisfactory experience in hospital are more likely to seek a home birth next time and vice versa for those who did not like home birth. Given that the number of women having planned home births is now so small, however, there is likely to be a greater proportion who are disenchanted with hospital delivery relative to the proportion of women giving birth in hospital who did not like home delivery.

In spite of the fact that in the last decade very few women have actually achieved a home delivery, demand for birth in places other than the obstetric unit seems to be surprisingly high. In a study of a cohort of 1000 consecutive births in one London maternity hospital (Morgan *et al* 1984) women were sent a questionnaire one year after delivery. The researchers claimed that the survey results were based on 'a large and representative group of mothers' and showed that 'women spurned home delivery'. Such a claim is rather misleading. A survey of the views of women delivering at one London hospital, to which slightly less than two thirds responded, cannot be considered truly representative. Moreover, only just over half (54 per cent) of those who responded actually disagreed with the statement 'Home deliveries ought to be encouraged'. Of the remainder 30 per cent neither agreed nor disagreed and 16 per cent agreed with it.

Renée Short, chair of the Social Services Committee during the time of its enquiry into perinatal and neonatal mortality, labelled those women who wanted home births as a lot of 'fuddy duddy middle class mothers' (Gillie 1980). Certainly there is evidence showing that a disproportionate number of women having planned home births are middle class (Campbell *et al* 1984), but research indicates that there is a demand for this form of delivery from women of all social backgrounds (Shepperdson 1983). Estimates from a variety of sources (Campbell 1979; Morgan *et al* 1984; Taylor 1986; Holdsworth 1989) suggest that between 10 and 15 per cent of women would like to give birth at home, which in England and Wales would mean something in the region of 66 000 to 99 000 births per annum.

■ General practitioner maternity care

The relationship between GP maternity care and place of birth is not straightforward. GPs do not provide intrapartum care in one particular place of birth but may provide it in a GP bed within a consultant unit, in a GP unit on a hospital site with consultant obstetric facilities, in an isolated GP unit or at home. As with home births there has been controversy over the safety and cost effectiveness of isolated GP maternity units; thus, it is this particular place of birth on which this section will focus.

Birth registration statistics identify separately births which take place in hospitals which have no consultant obstetric unit. These 'NHS A' hospitals, as they are classified, are of course what are more generally termed isolated GP units. Published data from the 'linked file' shown in Table 1.2 indicate that the proportion of births taking place in these units has dropped considerably in the last 11 years. Only low risk women are normally booked for delivery in these units so, as might be expected, the level of perinatal mortality compares very favourably with the overall rate. Interestingly however, data published for 1986 included, for the first time, birthweight specific perinatal mortality rates by place of birth. These showed that perinatal mortality rates for babies born in isolated GP units weighing 2500 grams or more and those of a low birth weight are significantly lower than these rates for all births (OPCS Monitor 1988). These data however do not paint the full picture as they do not include women booked for this form of care but transferred to consultant units either during pregnancy or labour.

A number of recent studies (Cavenagh *et al* 1984; Garrett *et al* 1987; Young 1987) have indicated however that even when transfers in labour are taken into account very low rates of perinatal mortality can be achieved. The findings of these studies are shown in Table 1.3. While these results indicate the risk of perinatal death associated with actual and intended delivery in an isolated GP unit, there has been no attempt to control for the selection biases which arise because only low risk women are booked for this form of care in the first place. A number of studies have attempted to control for this type of bias by comparing similar groups of low risk women delivering under different forms of care. An example of this type of study was that undertaken by Taylor and colleagues (1980) in which the delivery outcomes for low risk women giving birth in one health authority where 34 per cent of births took place in isolated GP units, were compared with deliveries in two other areas where there were no GP units. No statistically significant differences were found between perinatal mortality rates for the three areas. These findings were supported by the results of a later study in

Table 1.2 Perinatal mortality rates (PNMRs) for all births and babies born in isolated general practitioner units, (IGPUs) England and Wales, 1975–1986

Year	Number of births in IGPUs	Births in IGPUs as a percentage of all births	Number of perinatal deaths in IGPUs	PNMR per 1000 births	Total number of perinatal deaths	PNMR per 1000 births
1975	43862	7.2	218	5.0	11716	19.2
1976	45458	7.7	191	4.2	10416	17.7
1977	39019	6.8	202	5.2	9717	16.9
1978	35645	5.9	179	4.9	9313	15.5
1979	32700	5.1	122	3.7	9402	14.6
1980	27225	4.1	101	3.7	8796	13.3
1981	22210	3.5	63	2.8	7521	11.8
1982	21056	3.3	42	2.0	7060	11.2
1983	16694	3.1	41	2.1	6561	10.4
1984	18435	2.9	37	2.0	6440	10.1
1985	16346	2.5	27	1.6	6463	9.8
1986	14907	2.2	35	2.3	6338	9.5

Source: OPCS Birth statistics, Series FM1 and Mortality Statistics, Series DH3

another health authority (Black 1982) which 'failed to show that a high proportion of general practitioner deliveries constituted a major perinatal risk'.

Michael Klein and Luke Zander (1989) have recently undertaken a review of all the published studies which have compared the outcome of intrapartum care provided by GP with that provided by obstetricians. In only one study from the United States (Caetano 1975) did they find evidence that GP care was associated with poorer outcomes. The author of this study reported more birth injuries in the population cared for by family practitioners. All the other studies reviewed indicated that outcomes were similar for both forms of care.

In addition to evidence that GPs can provide safe maternity care for low risk women there is evidence that women prefer this type of care. A recent postal survey of 756 women who gave birth in the Bath Health District over a two month period (Taylor 1986) showed that women preferred ante- and postnatal care to be provided by a GP. Of the 562 women who responded, 64 per cent indicated that for a subsequent birth, providing everything was normal, they would prefer a GP delivery in hospital. Of the remainder, 12 per cent said they would like a home delivery and 25 per cent expressed a preference for consultant care. Women were also asked about their preferences if there was a slight risk of something going wrong. Under these

Table 1.3   Perinatal mortality rates for births occurring and intended to occur in isolated GP units (IGPU)

Study details			Perinatal mortality per 1000 births	
Year(s) study carried out	Authors	Location	Birth in IGPU	IGPU intended place of birth
1982	Cavenagh *et al*	England & Wales	1.1*	5.2*
1980–1984	Young	Penrith	0.87	4.7
1978–1985	Garrett *et al*	Bristol	1.7	1.5

* These rates are based on responses to a postal questionnaire from 116 out of 131 IGPUs in England and Wales.

circumstances 62 per cent said they would prefer consultant care, 37 per cent a GP delivery in hospital and only two per cent a home delivery.

■ Size of delivery units

The policy of closing small maternity units, be they consultant or GP units, has been pursued on the grounds of economy and greater safety. As with other aspects of policy on place of birth there is little scientific justification for this.

There is a growing body of evidence from a variety of countries (Hemminki 1985; Rosenblatt *et al* 1985; Lumley 1988) which suggests that babies of a normal birthweight do less well in larger hospitals. Only one study (Sax 1983) has found small hospitals to be associated with poorer perinatal outcomes.

Evidence on the outcomes of low birthweight infants is slightly less clear but, in a recent study, Lumley (1988) notes that when lethal malformations were excluded and late transfer included 'all low birthweight categories showed a significantly better outcome in the largest hospitals'. Lumley concludes that 'effective regionalisation need not involve the closure of small maternity units on the grounds of safety', but, 'because of the complexity of social, medical and geographical elements in the provision of perinatal care', she suggests that it is unwise to extrapolate the findings of her analysis of births in Victoria, Australia to other areas.

Although the argument that isolated GP units are not cost effective has been used to justify closure, there are remarkably few published economic appraisals of the costs of providing maternity care in different locations. Attempts to compare the costs of delivery in consultant units and GP units have produced somewhat contradictory findings. Ferster and Pethybridge (1973) found costs for women who delivered without intervention were lower for those giving birth in a consultant unit. In a similar study Gray and Steele (1981) found costs were lower for GP units but they made no attempt to control for the fact that deliveries in a consultant unit were likely to contain a higher proportion of complex cases requiring more expensive care. A recent review of this subject (Mugford 1988) found that, 'the case is not proven that GP maternity care is uneconomic. Indeed, the evidence points to the opposite conclusion'.

■ Recommendations for clinical practice in the light of currently available evidence

The scientific evidence relating to the place of birth suggests that:

- The temporal relationship between the increase in the proportion of births taking place in hospital and the decline in perinatal mortality is not one of cause and effect;

- Hospital may not always be the safest place in which to give birth;

- While not conclusive, morbidity for both mother and baby appears to be higher among deliveries in hospital;

- For women expected to have normal deliveries in hospital there is no difference in outcome whether the woman is under the care of a GP practitioner or a consultant obstetrician;

- Forms of maternity care other than those based on consultant obstetrics are not uneconomic;

- For low birthweight babies, delivery in a large obstetric unit does seem to be associated with an enhanced chance of survival but for normal birthweight babies the reverse seems to be true;

- Of those women who have experienced both home and hospital delivery the vast majority preferred giving birth at home;

- In spite of the policy towards delivery in large consultant units and the current lack of choice there is still a considerable demand for alternative forms of intrapartum care.

The following recommendations on place of birth, laid out by the Royal College of Midwives (1987) in the policy document 'Towards a healthy nation' (paragraph 4), provide an excellent guide for clinical practice.

1. Decisions on the place of confinement should be made on an individual basis with the parents in possession of full information.

2. A recognised home confinement service should exist in all health authorities and should be based on policy agreed by all relevant professionals.

3. A minority of women require the full range of hospital technology during childbirth. Techniques should be subject to continuous evaluation to help clarify their appropriate use for low and high risk groups of women.

4. Midwives should have full access to all facilities required for normal deliveries.

5. Maternity units should provide a range of delivery facilities to meet the various needs of all women through the spectrum of low to high risk.

6. Midwives as well as general practitioners and obstetricians, should have the right to admit clients to the hospital maternity unit.

7. All new maternity units should be on district general hospital sites so that the full range of back up services can be provided.

8. Treatment protocols should be agreed by all involved professionals working in a maternity unit and should provide a guide to current good practice.

9. Research into the value of continuous fetal heart monitoring for women with different risk factors should be undertaken.

10. Anyone who undertakes responsibility for a delivery should be able to initiate immediate resuscitation of the newborn. Equipment for this should be available at all deliveries including home deliveries.

11. The wishes of the family must be paramount when training experience for students is required.

12. Where stillbirth or neonatal death occurs a designated senior member of staff should take direct responsibility to ensure that parents receive full information and counselling.

■ Practice check

●· What are your own beliefs about the comparative safety of the home and hospital birth? Have they changed in the light of information contained in this chapter?

- What information or advice would you give to a woman who asks about a home birth?

- What do you currently tell pregnant women about the alternatives available to them?

- Find out what your local home delivery rate is and whether it has changed over recent years. If it has why is this?

- Have you ever been present at a home birth? If not might it be possible to rectify this?

- Investigate the composition of Midwifery Liaison Committees (and others) that are influential in formulating local maternity services policy such as that on place of birth. (These committees should contain midwives of all grades together with lay members and obstetricians.)

- Consider your own skills regarding the critical appraisal of research literature so that not every research report is accepted unquestioningly.

□ Acknowledgements

The author wishes to thank Alison Macfarlane of the National Perinatal Epidemiology Unit, Oxford, co-author of 'Where to be born? The debate and the evidence' from which parts of this chapter have been drawn.

Thanks are also due to Marjorie Tew for permission to reproduce the results of her analysis of data from the 1970 British Births Survey in Table 1.1, and to the Royal College of Midwives for permission to reproduce recommendations on place of birth from 'Towards a Healthy Nation'.

■ References

Alment E A J, Barr A, Reid M, Reid J J A 1967 Normal confinement: a domiciliary and hospital study. British Medical Journal 2: 530–35
Ashford J R 1978 Policies for maternity care in England and Wales: too fast too far? In: Kitzinger S, Davis J (eds) The place of birth. Oxford University Press, Oxford
Barron S L, Thomson A M, Philips P R 1977 Home and hospital confinement in Newcastle-upon-Tyne 1960–1969. British Journal of Obstetrics and Gynaecology 84: 401–11
Black N 1982 Do general practitioner deliveries constitute a perinatal mortality risk? British Medical Journal 284: 488–90
Brody H, Thompson J R 1981 The maximum strategy in modern obstetrics. Journal of Family Practice 12: 977–86

Butler N R, Alberman E D 1969 Perinatal problems. Livingstone, Edinburgh, London

Caetano D F 1975 The relationship of medical specialization (obstetricians and general practitioners) to complications in pregnancy and delivery, birth injury and malformation. American Journal of Obstetrics and Gynecology 123: 221–27

Campbell R 1979 A study of selected aspects of the change in the place of confinement with particular reference to Plymouth. Unpublished undergraduate dissertation, Plymouth Polytechnic

Campbell R, Macdonald Davies I, Macfarlane A 1982 Perinatal mortality and place of delivery. Population Trends 28: 9–12

Campbell R, Macdonald Davies I, Macfarlane A, Beral V 1984 Home births in England and Wales; perinatal mortality according to intended place of delivery. British Medical Journal 289: 721–24

Campbell R, Macfarlane A 1987 Where to be born? The debate and the evidence. National Perinatal Epidemiology Unit, Oxford

Caplan M, Madeley R J 1985 Home deliveries in Nottingham 1980–81. Public Health 99: 307–13

Cavenagh A J M, Phillips K M, Sheridan B, Williams E M J 1984 Contribution of isolated general practitioner maternity units. British Medical Journal 288: 1438–40

Chalmers I, Zlosnik J E, Johns K A, Campbell H 1976 Obstetric practice and outcome of pregnancy in Cardiff residents 1965–1973. British Medical Journal 1: 735–8

Chalmers I, Macfarlane A J 1980 Interpretation of perinatal statistics. In Wharton B (ed) Topics in perinatal medicine. Pitman, London

Chamberlain G, Phillip E, Howlett B, Masters K 1978 British Births 1970, Volume 2, Obstetric Care. Heinemann, London

Chamberlain R, Chamberlain G, Hewlett B, Claireaux A 1975 British births 1970, volume 1, the first week of life. Heinemann, London

Damstra-Wijmenga S M I 1984 Home confinement: the positive results in Holland. Journal of the Royal College of General Practitioners 34: 425–30

DHSS 1970 Domiciliary midwifery and maternity bed needs (Peel Report) HMSO, London

Ferster G, Pethybridge R 1973 The costs of a local maternity care system. Hospital and Health Services Review July: 243–47

Flint C, Poulengeris P, Grant A 1989 The 'Know Your Midwife scheme' – a randomised trial of continuity of care by a team of midwives. Midwifery 5: 11–16

Fryer J G, Ashford A 1972 Trends in perinatal and neonatal mortality in England and Wales 1960–9. British Journal of Preventive Social Medicine 26: 1–9

Garrett T, House W, Lowe S W 1987 Outcome of women booked into an isolated general practitioner maternity unit over eight years. Journal of the Royal College of General Practitioners 37: 488–90

Gillie O 1980 Hospital v home childbirth row looms. Sunday Times 16 November: 6

Gray A M, Steele R 1981 The economics of specialist and general practitioner maternity units. Journal of the Royal College of General Practitioners 31: 586–92

Goldthorpe W O, Richman J 1974 Maternal attitudes to unintended home confinements. A case study of the effects of a hospital strike upon domiciliary confinements. Practitioner 212: 845–53.

Gordon I, Elias Jones T F 1960 The place of confinement: home or hospital? The mother's preference. British Medical Journal 52: 3

Hansard 1987 House of Commons. Parliamentary Debates 121, col 910: W

Heady J A, Daly C, Morris J N 1955 Social and biological factors in infant mortality II. Variations of mortality with mother's age and parity. Lancet ii: 395–97

Heady J A, Morris J N 1956 Social and biological factors in infant mortality VI. Mothers who have their babies in hospitals and nursing homes. British Journal of Preventive Social Medicine 10: 97–106

Hemminki E 1985 Perinatal mortality distributed by type of hospital in the central hospital district of Helsinki, Finland. Scandinavian Journal of Social Medicine 13: 113–18

Holdsworth J 1989 The role of the general practitioner in intrapartum obstetric care. Unpublished General Practice project. Sheffield University Medical School

House of Commons Social Services Committee (HC) 1980 Perinatal and neonatal mortality. Second report from the Social Services Committee, Sessions 1979–80, Vol I: Cmnd. 663–I. HMSO, London

Hudson C K 1968 Domiciliary obstetrics in a groups practice. Practitioner 201: 816–22

James R 1977a Letter to New Society 39: 248

James D K 1977b Patients transferred in labour from general practitioner maternity units. Journal of the Royal College of General Practitioners 27: 414–18

Joint Committee of the Royal College of Obstetricians and Gynaecologists and the Population Investigation Committee 1948 Maternity in Great Britain. Oxford University Press, Oxford

Kitzinger S, Davis J A 1978 The Place of Birth. Oxford University Press, Oxford

Klein M, Lloyd I, Redman C, Bull M, Turnbull A C 1980 A comparison of a sample of low-risk women delivering in two systems of care – shared care (consultant team) and community care (integrated general practice [GP] unit). Paper presented at Pregnancy Care for the 1980s held at the Royal Society of Medicine, London

Klein M, Lloyd I, Redman C, Bull M Turnbull A C 1983 A comparison of low risk pregnant women booked for delivery in two systems of care. British Journal of Obstetrics and Gynaecology 90: 118–22

Klein M, Elbourne D, Lloyd I 1985 Booking for maternity care, a comparison of two systems. Occasional paper 31. RCGP, London

Klein M, Zander L 1989 Role of the family practitioner in maternity care. In Chalmers I, Enkin M, Kierse M (eds) Effective care in pregnancy and childbirth. Oxford University Press, Oxford

Lievaart M, de Jong P A 1982 Neonatal morbidity in deliveries conducted by midwives and gynaecologists. American Journal of Obstetrics and Gynecology 114: 376–86

Lilford R J 1987 Clinical experimentation in obstetrics. British Medical Journal 295: 1298–1300

Lumley J 1988 The safety of small maternity hospitals in Victoria 1982–84. Community Health studies. XII (4): 386–93

Macdonald Davies I 1980 Perinatal and infant death rates: social and biological factors. Population Trends 19: 19–21

Maternity Services Advisory Committee 1984 Maternity Care in Action Part II Care during childbirth (intrapartum care): a guide to good practice and a plan for action. HMSO, London

Mehl L E 1978 The outcome of home delivery: research in the United States. In Kitzinger S, Davis J A (eds) The place of birth. Oxford University Press, Oxford

Morgan B M, Bulpitt C, Clifton P, Lewis P J 1984 The consumers' attitude to obstetric care. British Journal of Obstetrics and Gynaecology 91: 624–8

Ministry of Health 1920 Annual Report of the Chief Medical Officer 1919–1920. HMSO, London

Mugford M 1988 Economies of scale and low risk maternity care: what is the evidence. Unpublished paper

Murphy J F, Dauncey M, Gray O P, Chalmers I 1984 Planned and unplanned deliveries at home: implications of a changing ratio. British Medical Journal 288: 1429–32

O'Brien M 1978 Home and hospital confinement: a comparison of the experiences of mothers having home and hospital confinements. Journal of the Royal College of General Practitioners 28: 460–66

OPCS Monitor 1988 Infant and perinatal mortality 1986: Birthweight, DH3 88/1. Government Statistical Service, London

Rees H G St M 1961 A domiciliary obstetric practice 1948–58. Journal of the Royal College of General Practitioners 4: 47–71

Rosenblatt R A, Deinken J, Shoemack P 1985 Is obstetrics safe in small hospitals? Evidence from New Zealand's Regionalised Perinatal System. Lancet ii: 429–31

Royal College of Midwives 1987 Towards a healthy nation. RCM, London

Rutter P 1964 Domiciliary midwifery – is it justifiable. Lancet ii: 1228–30

Sax S 1983 Report of the Commission of Inquiry into South Australian Hospitals. South Australian Health Commission, Adelaide

Scherjon S 1986 A comparison between the organisation of obstetrics in Denmark and the Netherlands. British Journal of Obstetrics and Gynaecology 93: 684–89

Schwarz E 1990 The engineering of childbirth: a new obstetric programme as reflected in British obstetric textbooks, 1960–1980. In: Garcia J, Kilpatrick R, Richards M (eds) The politics of maternity care. Oxford University Press, Oxford

Senn S J Unpublished analyses

Shaw G B S 1906 Preface to 'The Doctor's Dilemma'. Constable, London

Shearer J M L 1985 Five year prospective survey of risk of booking for home birth. British Medical Journal 291: 1478–80

Shepperdson B 1983 Home or hospital birth? A study of women's attitudes. Health Visitor 56: 405–6

Taylor A 1986 Maternity Services: the consumer's view. Journal of the Royal College of General Practitioners 36: 157–60

Taylor G W, Edgar W, Taylor B A, Neal D G 1980 How safe is general practitioner obstetrics? Lancet   ii: 1287–89

Tew M 1978 The case against hospital deliveries: the statistical evidence. In Kitzinger S, Davis J A (eds) The place of birth. Oxford University Press, Oxford

Tew M 1981 Effects of scientific obstetrics on perinatal mortality. Health and Social Services Journal   91: 444–46

Tew M 1985a Place of birth and perinatal mortality. Journal of the Royal College of General Practitioners   35: 390–4

Tew M 1985b Home births: we have the technology. Nursing Times   81 (47): 22–4

Tew M 1986 Do obstetric interventions make births safer? British Journal of Obstetrics and Gynaecology   93: 659–74

Tew M 1987 Is home birth less safe? Paper presented at the First International Conference on Home Birth, October 24th and 25th, Wembley Conference Centre, London

Treffers P E, Laan R 1986 Regional perinatal mortality and regional hospitalisation at delivery in the Netherlands. British Journal of Obstetrics and Gynaecology   93: 690–93

Woodall J 1968 No place like home. Proceedings of the Royal Society of Medicine   61: 1032–34

Young G 1987 Are isolated maternity units run by general practitioners dangerous? British Medical Journal   294: 744–46

■ Suggested further reading

Campbell R, Macfarlane A 1987 Where to be born? The debate and the evidence. National Perinatal Epidemiology Unit, Oxford

Tew M 1985 Place of birth and perinatal mortality. Journal of the Royal College of General Practitioners   35: 390–94

Garcia J, Kilpatrick R, Richards M P 1990 The politics of maternity care. Oxford University Press, Oxford

Klein M, Zander L 1989 The role of the family practitioner in maternity care. In Chalmers I, Enkins M, Kierse M (eds) Effective care in pregnancy and childbirth. Oxford University Press, Oxford

Chapter 2

Midwifery care in the first stage of labour

Sheila Drayton

> It was a marvellous experience. I had the very best treatment for myself, my husband and my baby. Ten out of ten for help and care.

> Now, six months after my labour, I still feel angry and distressed when I think about it. I have been left with an overwhelming sense of failure.
>
> (*Parents* magazine survey 1983)

The above quotations reflect the wide range of feelings expressed by mothers about their labours. This chapter is written with the intention of exploring the way in which good midwifery practice can contribute to a positive experience of labour for the mother, enabling her to enter parenthood with a sense of achievement and a degree of confidence. It is of course accepted that this outcome cannot be considered in isolation, and therefore the chapter begins by acknowledging that a safe outcome for the mother and baby is the primary objective of care in labour. Having established these two objectives, the chapter goes on to review current midwifery practice in the first stage of labour and the extent to which it contributes to these outcomes. In recent years admission procedures, including perineal shaving and the administration of enemas, have been criticised by consumer groups, and these will be considered in detail. At present, the organisation of maternity care in hospitals is being reviewed in many areas, and this chapter considers the way in which different patterns of care affect communication between the woman and those caring for her.

■ It is assumed that you are already aware of the following:

● The anatomy of the female genital tract;

● The physiology of labour;

- The guidelines or policies for the management of the first stage of labour in your unit or sphere of practice.

■ The desired outcomes of labour

Before considering current midwifery practice in the first stage of labour, it is important to establish the desired outcomes of labour, for it is against these objectives that we must measure midwifery practice. Only when the outcomes have been agreed can we critically evaluate present practice, and determine to what extent it contributes to, and is necessary for, achieving the desired outcomes of labour.

There is little doubt that mothers, midwives and obstetricians would agree that the most desirable outcome of labour is the safe delivery of a healthy, mature infant to a well mother. The rationale for this outcome is self evident. Every woman in labour wishes to be safely delivered of a healthy baby, and in the wider context a healthy infant will be better able to contribute to society.

The second most desirable outcome of labour is less well defined. Increasingly midwives and obstetricians are coming to recognise that labour should be a positive experience for the woman, enabling her to enter parenthood with a sense of achievement and a degree of confidence. The rationale for this outcome is that the future relationship between the mother and the infant is affected by the mother's feelings following delivery.

In 1989, Jean Ball found that women who expressed themselves as 'disappointed', or 'too tired to care' following delivery, scored 'significantly lower levels of satisfaction with motherhood six weeks after delivery'. In contrast, those who described themselves as 'gloriously happy' at delivery, showed 'very much higher satisfaction with motherhood six weeks later'. Her study also showed that satisfaction with motherhood 'had a positive effect upon emotional well being, boosting morale and enriching the adjustment process' (Ball 1989).

The benefits of a positive experience of delivery are linked, therefore, to satisfaction with motherhood, which in turn has a positive effect on emotional wellbeing and enriches the adjustment process. This provides a favourable foundation for the development of the mother-child relationship.

Less well documented is the adverse effect a bad experience of labour can have on women. The evidence for this is mainly anecdotal, but given so frequently, that it is worthy of consideration. It is usually provided by women who retain bitter feelings about care in labour for many years. Most midwives will be familiar with the situation which can occur in the social context if it is disclosed that the listener is a midwife. The author remembers listening to a particularly harrowing story related by a woman to whom she had just been introduced. This woman quoted the exact words of the midwife in every detail. It was the story of the birth of her son and it concerned care rather than a life and death situation, but it distressed her greatly. She concluded by saying. 'Of course, he is 25 years old now'. I was shocked. It was clear that time had in no way dimmed her memory of what she regarded as her humiliation and failure, and the midwife's hostile attitude. It cannot be determined whether this experience influenced the woman's life or affected her relationship with her son, but it remained very vivid to her.

The story serves as a reminder of the awesome responsibility that midwives bear, especially during labour, for even their most casual remarks are likely to be recalled and mulled over for many years.

It must be remembered then, that women in labour are about to assume the responsibility of parenthood, and the experience of labour should do nothing to diminish their confidence; instead, it should promote a sense of achievement, ability and preparedness.

The achievement of satisfaction with 'self' and the service is sometimes described as a 'soft' outcome. And it is accepted that where conflict arises between the 'hard' outcome of a live infant and a live mother, and the 'soft' outcome of satisfaction, the former will take precedence. Care must be taken however not to allow the achievement of a safe outcome to become an excuse for neglecting the needs of women.

In conclusion then, the desired outcomes of labour are:

- A safe outcome for mother and baby;
- A positive experience of labour for the woman.

■ Achieving the outcomes

□ A safe outcome for mother and baby

It is intended to give only an overview of the principal methods of achieving a safe outcome for mother and baby. These are monitoring the normal progress of labour, detecting deviations from the normal, and intervening appropriately if deviations from the normal occur.

□ Monitoring the normal progress of labour

This refers to the following:

- Monitoring the wellbeing of the infant – by noting the fetal heart rate and rhythm, and/or the cardiotocograph trace;

- Monitoring the wellbeing of the mother – by noting her psychological wellbeing, her blood pressure, pulse and temperature, and by testing her urine for the presence of protein or ketones;

- Monitoring the progress of labour which is indicated by descent of the presenting part, dilatation of the cervix, and the increase in the strength, length and frequency of contractions.

☐ **Detecting deviations from the normal**

Deviations from the normal should be detected using the criteria above.

☐ **Intervening appropriately if deviations from the normal occur**

Examples of interventions will include:

- Restoring maternal and fetal wellbeing by giving nourishing fluids or an intravenous infusion;

- Accelerating labour;

- Delivering the infant by caesarean section.

During the last two decades, the majority of obstetricians in the Western world have come to believe that monitoring the wellbeing of the infant and to a lesser extent the wellbeing of the mother during labour, can best be achieved with the use of sophisticated medical technology. This view is questioned in the literature (Banta & Thecker 1979), but further discussion of the relative value of medical technology in obstetrics is outside the remit of this chapter. Suffice it to say that electronic fetal heart monitoring has become an integral part of the care of women in labour in most major maternity units. This has led to an increased emphasis on the physical management of the woman and her baby, possibly to the exclusion of the psychological care of the woman. Where this imbalance has occured, it needs to be redressed.

☐ **A positive experience of labour for the woman**

This outcome is about enabling the woman to retain her persona and her dignity, and about enabling her to maintain and enhance her confidence in herself. In order to achieve this she needs to understand events and participate in decisions about her labour. This means feeling able to ask questions and communicate with her midwife and with others. There may be difficulties here however. Good communication is the outcome of a two way process between equals, and there is ample evidence that women in labour do not feel equal and have difficulty in obtaining information (Cartwright 1979; Oakley 1979; Kirke 1980). It follows that the way to assist a woman to achieve a positive experience of childbirth is to empower her so that she will be able to ask questions, understand events and participate in decisions about her care.

■ Midwifery practice – contributing to positive outcomes?

Having established the desired outcomes of labour and the methods of achieving the outcomes, we can now move on to consider current midwifery practice in the first stage of labour. By critically appraising the research literature we will determine to what extent it contributes to a safe outcome and a positive experience of labour.

Three aspects of practice will be studied in detail. These are:

● The admission procedure and information giving;

● Preparation for labour, including perineal shaving and bowel preparation;

● Communication and the organisation of care within maternity units.

■ Admission – the beginning of a partnership or putting the woman in the patient role

Discussion of this subject will be based primarily on two studies. The first was carried out by Mavis Kirkham (1989) and is a qualitative, descriptive study of 113 labours. Kirkham observed 90 of the labours in the consultant unit of a Northern teaching hospital, five were home confinements and 18 took place in a general practitioner maternity unit. The second study (Garforth & Garcia 1987) was designed to examine routines in midwifery care. The study had two stages – a postal survey of Directors of Midwifery Services, followed by an in-depth study of aspects of policy and practice in eight health districts, during which 62 admissions of women in normal labour were observed.

Garforth and Garcia noted that the midwife may have different priorities to those of the women during the admission procedure, confirming the findings of Kirkham (1983).

A woman entering hospital at the end of her pregnancy is unlikely to feel at home in the building and is unlikely to know the midwife who is admitting her. So she needs to orientate herself within the unit and to establish relationships with those caring for her. She may be feeling extremely vulnerable, particularly if this is her first baby. At the same time, she is experiencing physiological changes which are both exciting, since they herald the birth of her baby, and a cause of anxiety because she may not understand the changes fully and has little control over them. She needs to know whether all is well and to find out how her labour is likely to progress.

The midwife meanwhile, needs to make a clinical assessment of the wellbeing of the mother and the infant, and of the progress of labour. She also has to complete a number of forms and record her findings, and she may be required to 'prep' the woman by ensuring that the woman's bowel, puboperineal area and skin are prepared for labour in accordance with local guidelines.

Whilst these two sets of priorities are not mutually exclusive, there is evidence that frequently the interaction between the midwife and the woman during the admission procedure is dominated by the need to complete forms and preparation procedures. This militates against the woman achieving her objectives of obtaining information and establishing a relationship with her carers.

Kirkham (1989) found that form filling starts early in the admission process, and usually begins with the question, 'when did your contractions become regular'. Women often give lengthy replies, describing the circumstances and the sensations of early labour, but the form requires a short, precise answer. As Kirkham notes, 'the midwife usually filled it in with a brief remark such as: "I'll put 4.30." After that, the woman's replies typically become much shorter.'

The woman realises that her detailed view of events is neither needed nor valued. This is unlikely to enhance her confidence, or encourage her to ask the questions which will enable her to meet her objectives.

Kirkham (1983) also observed that if questions are asked, they are frequently met with such phrases as 'Don't worry', or 'Relax, you're in the right place'. These responses do not provide the information the woman needs, so her worries remain. Instead, the responses serve to reinforce the notion that she should not seek to understand and participate, but should leave the management of labour to the midwife.

A tendency to treat women in a similar way to children was also found by Garforth and Garcia (1987). They observed the initial contact between the mother and the midwife on 36 occasions. Only seven midwives asked the woman what she would like to be called. The other midwives fell into three categories: 'Some assumed that the woman did not mind being called by her first name; some remained on a formal basis using "Mrs", while others adopted some more familiar terms such as "lovey" or "pet"'. The researchers quote a woman who said, 'I don't like being called "lovey" ... it made me feel as if I was a child'. They also note that midwives frequently used the phrase 'Good girl'.

In the same study, Garcia and Garforth noted that in 23 per cent of the cases observed, midwives did not take the opportunity during admission to discuss the woman's preferences or plans for labour. Clearly, here was an opportunity to establish a relationship, but it was missed. The midwives were better at explaining what they were doing however; 43 out of 49 gave either excellent, good or quite good explanations, but the emphasis was on what was happening rather than why. If women are to understand events and participate in their care, they need to know why.

☐ **Companions, undressing and privacy**

Mavis Kirkham (1983) has suggested that not only in our words, but also in our actions, we may be stripping the woman of her identity and reducing her to being a 'patient' who is easy to manage. This we achieve by stripping her 'of her next of kin, her clothes, her pubic hair and the contents of her bowel'.

These are emotive words and much has changed since 1983, but change has not been universal or uniform.

Garforth and Garcia (1987) found that in four of the districts studied, it was routine practice for the partner to be included in the admission procedure, whereas in the other four districts he was usually excluded. The midwives' comments in the districts encouraging partners included:

Yes for admission they are encouraged, there are no restrictions now. They can have parents or other relatives.

It's the Mum's choice. There are no exceptions.

The researchers were told by some of the midwives in the districts where partners were usually excluded that partners could have stayed if they had wished. In many of the observed cases, however, the study found that partners were asked to wait as a matter of course, without being given any real choice.

When the women were interviewed, only 3 per cent preferred not to have anyone with them at admission. Those whose partners were unable to stay were disappointed. Garforth and Garcia quote the following comments:

I was upset. I think you need someone who knows you.

I would have liked him to be with me, but they told him to wait. He wanted to come in, but did not say anything, although we had talked about it at home.

Soon after arrival in the maternity unit, women in labour are asked to undress. Readers who have visited a hospital and been asked to take their day clothes off will appreciate that undressing immediately reduces one's sense of 'wholeness' and equality. This is exacerbated in maternity units if the woman is not able to secure her privacy whilst changing by shutting a door, and if the gown she is given is inadequate.

Garforth and Garcia quote the following midwife's instruction: 'Just take all your clothes off and pop on the bed. What buttons there are go down the front and you'll find there's a slit up the back'. It is worth reflecting on the effect such an instruction would have on one's own confidence.

Six of the districts in this study provided hospital gowns, but two asked women to bring in an old nightie of their own, and this appeared popular.

Provision for privacy was also found to be unsatisfactory, 'often involving curtains and screens of various designs, rather than a door which could be closed'.

From this review of the research on the admission of women in labour, we can conclude that the midwife and the woman may have differing priorities. The midwife must assess the woman's wellbeing and progress in labour, and indeed her assessment contributes to a safe outcome for the mother and infant. At the same time the woman needs to be received in such a way that she feels she is a valued partner in her care. The evidence appears to show, however, that much of our admission behaviour seems likely to diminish the woman's sense of worth rather than to enhance it. Clearly there is a need to examine our practice, and to balance the priorities of the midwife and the woman so that we can contribute to a positive experience of labour as well as a safe outcome.

■ Preparation for labour

One has to begin by asking who or what are we preparing for labour? Is it the woman herself, in which case preparation would be concerned with meeting her needs as described in the previous section, or is it the woman's body that we are preparing for labour in isolation from the woman?

Preparation procedures for women in labour have a long history. Garforth and Garcia (1987) quote a description of the admission procedure in a New York hospital in the early 1900s (Mahan & McKay 1983). It included pubic shaving and an enema – as might be expected – but, in addition, women could expect their nipples and navel to be doused with ether and their heads to be cleansed with kerosene. Fortunately, the ether and kerosene were discontinued some time ago, but it is probably fair to say that pubic shaving and preparatory enemas became part of an almost hallowed tradition in maternity units.

□ Perineal shaving

Mona Romney (1982) notes with interest that the technique of perineal shaving was first described in 1904, the same year that Mr Gillette received a US patent on his safety razor. She tells us that he appears to have marketed it aggressively by employing travelling nurses to demonstrate its advantages. The claim was that perineal shaving reduced infection and facilitated suturing should it be necessary.

Romney informs us that as early as 1922 this claim was challenged by the findings of a study by Johnston and Sidall. They allocated 389 women alternately to shave and non-shave groups, and found that the incidence of puerperal fever was slightly higher in women who had been shaved. But as Romney reports, 'their findings were drowned in the flood of publicity by Mr Gillette and his company'. There is a lesson here.

Much later, in 1980, Romney was able to compare women receiving no shave, a partial shave and a complete shave. She found that there was no significant difference in the infection rates, and drew attention to the abrasions and discomforts caused by shaving. In her study, 98 per cent of the 453 women shaved were disappointed that they had been shaved. Oakley (1979) has also recorded women's concerns about shaving.

From the evidence, we can conclude that shaving cannot be shown to contribute to a safe outcome, and it is likely to cause discomfort and abrasions. Furthermore, there is evidence that it is disliked by women and therefore it militates against a positive experience of labour. Therefore one would expect the practice to be discontinued. Although there has been a marked reduction in the number of women shaved from nine out of ten in 1981, to less than three out of ten in 1986 (Parents magazine survey 1986), shaving policy still remains very variable. Garforth and Garcia (1987) found that in more than half the consultant units in their study a proportion of women were shaved.

Why does the practice persist? Perhaps there are some midwives and obstetricians who continue to share the views of Margaret Myles (1972), 'that the majority of midwives prefer shaving to be done and many think that patients objections have been exaggerated'. Myles did not, of course, have access to Romney's (1980) work, but today's midwives do.

□ Enemas

The practice of administering enemas has a much longer history than shaving. Romney (1982) describes its origins in Ancient Egypt and traces its development in all the major civilisations of the world. She notes that enemas were very popular in the reign of Louis XIV and aristocratic women would have as many as three or four a day, however pregnant women were advised to reduce the amount of fluid as pregnancy progressed.

During this century enemas have been administered routinely to women in labour. It was held that an enema reduced the length of labour by reflexly stimulating uterine action, reduced faecal contamination of the delivery area and therefore reduced the risk of infection to mother and baby.

The use of enemas in delivery was questioned by Romney and Gordon in 1981. They suggested there was little evidence to support the continuation of what was a traditional part of delivery. Despite their work, enemas remained a common feature of delivery in many maternity units. A further study (Drayton & Rees 1989) was designed to replicate Romney and Gordon's (1981) work. The method differed from that of the previous authors who, because of initial resistance from staff, found it difficult to design an effective protocol for the trial. By now attitudes were changing and it was possible to carry out a randomised contolled trial to test three hypotheses. These were that an enema:

- Reduces the length of labour;
- Reduces faecal contamination of the delivery area;
- Reduces the risk of infection to mother and baby.

The second part of the study was designed to record how women themselves felt about the administration of enemas. The enema used in the study was a low volume disposable phosphate enema.

All women admitted for vaginal delivery with single pregnancies of 37 weeks or more gestation were eligible for inclusion in the study. Those excluded were women with medical conditions such as diabetes mellitus, heart disease and women with complications of pregnancy such as antepartum haemorrhage and severe pregnancy induced hypertension.

The study took place over a 10 week period during which 370 women satisfied the inclusion criteria and progressed to vaginal delivery. Of these, 222 agreed to enter the trial, and 148 declined. Among those declining, only 23 per cent chose to have an enema, which suggests that when given a choice, the majority of women will choose delivery without an enema. The results which follow are based on the study population of 222 women.

☐ **Duration of labour**

Duration of labour was measured in two hour segments ranging from under four hours to twelve hours plus. The results were compared for each parity group, but there was no significant difference in the length of labour for the enema and no enema groups.

The results do not support the hypothesis that an enema reduces the length of labour. This is an important statement, as it is perhaps the most commonly expressed 'belief' surrounding the use of enemas.

☐ **Soiling**

To measure the level of soiling, Drayton and Rees used the following four point scale in which 0 = clean; 1 = minimal faecal soiling; 2 = no more than two formed motions or episodes of diarrhoea; 3 = frequent formed or fluid motions. This scale had been used by Romney and Gordon (1981), and was found to be acceptable and easy to use during the pilot study. The midwife conducting the delivery was asked to record the level of soiling separately for each stage of labour.

The first stage results were similar to previous studies with less than 15 per cent of women in each group contaminating the delivery area. In the second stage, the expulsive efforts of the woman led to an increase in soiling in both groups. The increase was highest in the no enema group, with 45 per cent of women soiling compared to 22 per cent in the enema group. It is important, however, to note that the level of soiling for most of the women in the no enema group was in the minimal soiling category, and in the majority of cases the small amount of faecal matter was formed and easy to remove. This appears to be entirely acceptable to most midwives. This statement can be made with some accuracy, because following the study, the midwives did not resume the practice of giving enemas.

☐ **The problem of fluid soiling**

The type of soiling has been discussed by other authors. Whitley and Mack (1980) in a study in the USA, suggested that a small amount of liquid soiling was manageable. Romney and Gordon (1981) were of the opinion, however, that fluid soiling was more difficult to control. It was therefore decided to quantify the type of soiling that occurred.

In the Drayton and Rees (1989) study, fluid soiling occurred in over 50 per cent of the enema group in the first stage of labour, compared to none in the no enema group. In the second stage, the contrast was again well marked, with 50 per cent fluid soiling in the enema group and only 10 per cent in the no enema group. Therefore if fluid soiling is regarded as a problem, it can be shown that an enema greatly increases it. The midwives in the study found that fluid soiling contaminated more of the delivery area and shared the view that it was more difficult to control.

☐ **Infection**

All mothers and babies were monitored for signs of infection occurring within seven days of delivery. This was achieved with the help of a microbiologist, and a research midwife together with the senior sisters and community midwives. Infection was confirmed in 13 babies in the study; seven were in the no enema group, and six were in the enema group. One infant in each group had an umbilical infection, which could be related to bowel organisms (*streptoccus faecalis* and *E.coli* respectively). None of the mothers had a perineal wound infection.

This result is important, because it demonstrates that although the incidence of soiling in those women who did not receive an enema is higher, it is not associated with an increase in the infection rate. Therefore the third hypothesis that an enema reduces the risk of infection in the mother and baby can be rejected.

☐ **Women's views**

In the second part of the study women in both groups were asked how they felt about enemas. The results of this part of the study have been discussed more fully elsewhere (Drayton & Rees 1989), but some of the key points are given below.

It was found that for a number of women having their first baby the thought of receiving an enema was more frightening than the actual delivery. A great deal of anticipatory anxiety is thus evoked by a regimen of routine enemas. When asked to describe the experience of having an enema, those who had received one tended to use terms of discomfort and physical unpleasantness.

Clearly if enemas cause anticipatory anxiety and are associated with feelings of discomfort and physical unpleasantness, they will detract from a positive experience of labour. Therefore their continued use could only be justified if they contributed to a safe outcome of labour. The results of the clinical part of the study have shown that this is not so. It follows that a more personalised approach to this area of delivery should be adopted, with care plans tailored to meet the needs of individual women. The options will be discussed in the recommendations for clinical practice (see page 36).

■ The organisation of care – a cast of thousands?

Not very long ago we received a very fulsome 'thank you' letter from one of our clients. In her letter she expressed her gratitude to one or two midwives by name, and then to 'the cast of thousands' (her inverted commas), who had cared for her during her pregnancy and confinement. She was a confident, capable multigravid client who had clearly managed all of the 'getting to know you hurdles' that our pattern of care required.

At that time women in early labour were admitted to an antenatal ward where they would meet one group of staff. As labour progressed they were transfered to the labour ward where they would be cared for by a different team and finally following delivery, they would be taken to the postnatal ward, and yet another team. The author's personal feeling was that our grateful client had enjoyed a positive experience of labour in spite of us, and that less confident women might find it more difficult to repeatedly reorientate themselves and establish relationships with midwives and others.

There is some evidence to support this view. McIntosh (1988) found that lack of communication was a major source of complaint. Women complained that they were kept in the dark and this exacerbated their anxieties. At the same time it was noted that the majority of those 'who experienced difficulty with communication did not ask for information'. Similar results were obtained by Kirke (1980) in his study of 210 women. At least three quarters of the women desired more information but none of them asked the staff.

Earlier in this chapter we noted that women need to be empowered in order to feel confident and ask questions. A fragmented pattern of care, in which women are moved from one ward to another and from one group of staff to another must be seen as a serious obstacle to the establishment of good relationships and good communication.

The need for women to build up a relationship of trust with the staff they meet was recognised by The Maternity Services Advisory Committee in 1982. This report referred to the need for continuity of care in the antenatal period. Since then there has been a growing acceptance that, 'ideally', women should have the same midwife to attend them in labour as in the antenatal period. This has been achieved for a limited number of women, by small teams of midwives working in such schemes as the 'Know Your Midwife Scheme' (Flint & Poulgeneris 1987), and this must be the ultimate goal for all women. For the present, however, the majority of women are cared for in labour by midwives they may not have met, and in surroundings they may have visited only once if at all. We have noted the need for women to orientate themselves and to establish relationships with their carers. It follows that every effort should be made to ensure that they only have to do this once during their hospital stay. The ways in which this can be achieved will be discussed in the recommendations for clinical practice below.

■ Recommendations for clinical practice in the light of currently available evidence

Midwives should seek to empower women in their care. This will enable the women to feel confident, ask questions, understand events and participate in decisions about their labour. Ideally the woman should meet the midwife who will care for her in labour during the antenatal period. If this is not possible, she should be admitted and cared for in labour by one midwife who acts as the primary midwife, only transfering care if there is a change of shift.

☐ **Admission**

It is important to remember that every woman feels a degree of anxiety when she arrives at the hospital. Welcome her, introduce yourself in the way that you prefer to be known and demonstrate mutal respect by asking how she would like to be addressed. Avoid terms of endearment, they contribute to an unequal relationship.

You will need to make a clinical assessment but ensure that your interaction isn't dominated by form filling. Listen to the answers to your questions, taking care not to curtail responses. By valuing her answers, you will enhance her confidence. Try to encourage questions at this point for you will need to know her expectations if you are to develop a relationship of trust and understanding. Following your examination say something about progress thus far and something about the probable length of labour. This is the key question in every woman's mind and therefore it should not be avoided. Explain that it is often difficult to predict the length of labour with accuracy and indicate that you will update your estimate as labour progresses.

If the partner is present, remember that he may feel more anxious than the woman herself. Value his answers too and do not exclude him by word or tone. Try to give him real choice about remaining, if necessary, by saying that some partners choose to stay and others prefer to leave. Some couples welcome the confirmation that it is 'normal' for the partner to want to leave.

Where the plan for labour has already been prepared during the antenatal period it should be reviewed to ensure that both you and the client have a common understanding of the plan. If care in labour hasn't been discussed, try to introduce choice in a way which isn't worrying. Remember that some women may feel anxious if asked if they have thought about an alternative position for childbirth. At the same time others might wish to discuss alternatives, but not feel able to do so. A useful way of overcoming this difficulty is to ask if they have read or heard anything recently about ways of giving birth. The response to this question usually gives a clear indication of whether they wish to pursue the subject further.

☐ **Preparation for labour**

From the review of the literature it is clear that women must be enabled to retain their dignity during the admission procedure. They must be afforded privacy whilst changing, and they should be encouraged to use their own nightgown or be provided with an adequate hospital gown.

The practice of shaving either the puboperineal area or the perineal area should be discontinued. It does not contribute to a safer outcome, it causes abrasions and it is disliked by women.

Similarly the practice of routinely administering enemas to women in labour cannot be justified. In some countries it is the practice to ask women to open their bowels during the early part of the first stage of labour. This becomes a realistic option where women are afforded privacy, and it is recommended if the client has not moved her bowels within the last 12 to 24 hours. Failure to move the bowel is not catastrophic. In most cases it leads to a minimal amount of formed stool being passed during the second stage of labour which is easily removed. In some units suppositories are used, but this is again an invasive procedure, and there is no evidence to show that suppositories prevent a small amount of formed stool being passed in the second stage of labour. The problem of the loaded bowel requires further research. Drayton and Rees (1989) showed that the low volume disposable enema does not reduce soiling in the small group of women with a loaded bowel and therefore no firm recommendation for practice can be offered. The adoption of a more personalised approach to bowel preparation with care tailored to individual's needs will, however, benefit all clients.

☐ **Organisation of care**

In order to empower women they must be enabled to develop a trusting relationship with their midwife. Therefore hospital care must be arranged in a way which avoids changing carers and moving around from one ward to another. There is no longer the need for a separate admission room. Ideally women should be admitted to a delivery bedroom with an adjoining shower and toilet. The bedroom should be situated on the ward and if the woman is in early labour she will benefit from meeting the other women in the day room. Providing there are no complications in labour she will deliver in the delivery bedroom and then be taken or walk to her postnatal bed. The midwifery care ward therefore provides total care, and the woman retains her primary midwife.

Should complications arise in labour it may be necessary to transfer the woman to the labour ward, but whenever possible her midwife accompanies her.

In the absence of midwifery care wards, women should be admitted to comfortable rooms on the labour ward, where they should be cared for by their midwife.

It is sometimes difficult to bring about changes in the pattern of care, but increasingly midwifery managers are succeeding in negotiating improvements in the interests of the women they serve. Therefore we should not lower our sights but continue to press for a more holistic approach to maternity care.

■ Practice check

- What were the first words you said to the woman you admitted most recently?

- Did you ask her how she wished to be addressed?

- Did you use a term of endearment, such as 'pet' or 'dear'?

- Do you use the same term of endearment for all women?

- Did you curtail the woman's explanation of events? If yes, can you say why?

- Did you sit down to talk to her?

- Did you encourage participation by asking open questions such as, 'How do you feel about...?'

- Have any of your clients said 'sorry' or made remarks (such as 'I am a baby') which lower their status? If the answer is 'yes', you will need to reassess the way in which you are trying to achieve an equal partnership.

- Have you said 'don't worry' in response to a question this week? Remember women need real information not 'reassurance'.

- Do you allow women to undress in privacy without interruption? Do you and your colleagues knock before entering?

- What proportion of your clients are given perineal shaves? How does this compare with your colleagues' practice?

- What proportion of your clients are given an enema or suppository? How does this compare with the practice in other units?

- Does the pattern of care in your unit avoid moving women from ward to ward, and from midwife to midwife? If not, are you trying to influence managers in favour of change?

■ References

Ball J 1989 Postnatal care and adjustment to motherhood. In Robinson S, Thomson A (eds) Midwives, research and childbirth. Chapman and Hall, London

Banta H D, Thecker S B 1979 Costs and benefits of electronic fetal monitoring: a review of the literature. US Department of Health Education and Welfare, Washington DC

Cartwright A 1979 The dignity of labour: 114. Tavistock Publications, London

Drayton S M, Rees C 1989 Is anyone out there still giving enemas? In Robinson S, Thomson A (eds) Midwives, research and childbirth. Chapman and Hall, London

Flint C, Poulgeneris P 1987 The 'Know your midwife' report. Privately printed; available from 49 Peckarmans Wood, Sydenham Hill, London SE26 6RZ

Garforth S, Garcia J 1987 Admitting a weakness or a strength? Midwifery 3: 10–24

Johnston R A, Siddal R S 1922 Is the usual method of preparing patients for delivery beneficial or necessary? American Journal of Obstetrics and Gynecology 25: 509–12

Kirke P N 1980 Mothers' views of obstetric care. British Journal of Obstetrics and Gynaecology 87: 1029–33

Kirkham M 1983 Admission in labour: teaching the patient to be patient. Midwives Chronicle 96(2): 44–5

Kirkham M 1989 Midwives and information giving in labour. In Robinson S, Thomson A (eds) Midwives, research and childbirth. Chapman Hall, London

Maternity Services Advisory Committee 1982 Maternity care in action, Part I. Antenatal care. HMSO, London

McIntosh J 1988 Womens' views of communication in labour and delivery. Midwifery 4: 166–70

Mahan C S, McKay S 1983 Preps and enemas: keep or discard? Contemporary Obstetrics and Gynaecology 22(5): 173–84

Myles M F 1972 Textbook for Midwives, 7th ed.: 278. Churchill Livingstone, Edinburgh

Oakley A 1979 Becoming a mother. Martin Robertson, Oxford

Oakley A 1980 Women confined: towards a sociology of childbirth. Martin Robertson, Oxford

Parents magazine survey 1983 Birth in Britain. Parents 92: 13–16

Parents magazine survey 1986 Birth. Parents 128: 29–32

Romney M L 1980 Predelivery shaving: an unjustified assault? Journal of Obstetrics and Gynaecology 1: 33–5

Romney M L Gordon H 1981 Is your enema really necessary? British Medical Journal 282: 1269–71

Romney M L 1982 Nursing research in obstetrics and gynaecology. International Journal of Nursing Studies 19 (4): 193–203

Whitley N Mack E 1980 Are enemas justified for women in labour? American Journal of Nursing July: 1339

■ Suggested further reading

Drayton S M, Rees C 1989 Is anyone out there still giving enemas? In Robinson S, Thomson A (eds) Midwives, research and childbirth. Chapman and Hall, London

Garforth S, Garcia J 1987 Admitting a weakness or a strength?
    Midwifery   3: 10–24
Kirkham M, 1989 Midwives and information giving in labour. In Robinson S,
    Thomson A (eds) Midwives, research and childbirth. Chapman and Hall,
    London

Chapter 3

Artificial rupture of the membranes

Christine Henderson

Since the 1970s the management of childbirth has become more medicalised with greater dependency upon technology. Comaroff (1977) described midwives and obstetricians regarding childbirth as a condition similar to illness, suitably treated in terms of medical intervention and control, with pregnant women adopting a passive role. Chalmers and Richards, also writing in 1977, identified certain procedures as beneficial but pointed out that others carry risks to the mother and child and the benefit of *routine* usage was therefore doubtful. They made the following suggestions:

> a more rational framework for the evaluation of obstetric practice is needed: the quality of medical care depends on the extent to which interventions of proven effectiveness are properly applied to those who can benefit from them. Although there is nothing particularly novel about these views, there are grounds for believing that these principles are widely ignored (page 48).

The Association for the Improvement of Maternity Services (AIMS) continues to be concerned about the introduction of interventions prior to scientific evaluation and has recommended a government-led screening programme of all obstetric technologies.

In 1985, according to the World Health Organisation (WHO), the intervention rate in childbirth for Britain is higher than for other European countries. Birth was viewed as a mechanical process to be controlled, at any cost, rather than a biosocial event of great significance. Increasing control was advocated on the grounds of safety, but, today, many feel that the hospitalisation and increased technology furthers the self interest and satisfaction of obstetricians and aids them in assuming total control over what is, in most instances, a normal situation. These opinions are also expressed in the contributions collected by Kitzinger (1988), reflecting the state of midwifery/obstetric practice worldwide.

The movement for active management of labour has continued although there are differing views concerning its value when applied to all women irrespective of indication. Many professionals consider a 'short' labour to be beneficial; it is now common practice, therefore, to accelerate spontaneous labour by rupturing the membranes (amniotomy). This also enables observation of the baby's welfare while it is still *in utero* as the fetal heart can be monitored by attaching a fetal scalp electrode. In addition, it is argued that rupture of the membranes will enable any abnormality (for example meconium staining or deficiency in the amount of liquor) to be detected and appropriate action taken. Although artificial rupture of the membranes is an invasive procedure, the majority of midwives and obstetricians regard it as a straightforward, even insignificant, procedure which creates no problems, indeed as an accepted part of the management of childbirth. Women using the maternity services, however, continue to express concern over unnecessary interventions (Maternity Services Advisory Committee 1984; Jacoby 1987). Artificial rupture of the membranes, in itself, is a minor procedure but it raises certain questions about the mother's consent to treatment, her right to choose, and to decide how her labour is managed. Consequently it raises some important issues:

- Who should be involved in the decision-making process;

- Who should control the events surrounding childbirth;

- Who should take ultimate responsibility, the mother, the midwife, the obstetrician or all three?

This chapter has three main aims. The first of these is to describe the function of intact membranes and the process of rupture during normal labour. The second aim is to discuss the physiological and social issues surrounding artificial rupture of the membranes utilising the research available. Finally, the chapter will consider the implications for the midwife and midwifery practice.

■ It is assumed that you are already aware of the following:

- The physiology of labour;

- The policies and procedures regarding the management of labour in your own health authority;

- Satisfaction surveys completed by users of your own maternity services and/or the views of those using the service;

- How and who is involved in formulating a policy within your own health authority.

■ Rupture of the membranes in normal labour

Labour is the process by which the fetus, placenta and membranes are expelled from the uterus. Normal labour starts spontaneously between the 37th and 41st week culminating in the delivery of a live, healthy baby, placenta and membranes. The process is completed within 24 hours.

In normal labour the membranes rupture as a result of the force exerted by uterine contractions. Contractions originate in or near the cornua of the uterus, gradually spreading outwards and gaining most intensity on reaching the fundus. As labour progresses this degree of intensity becomes greater and more frequent increasing the fluid pressure within the amniotic cavity. The force exerted by the fundus during contractions is relayed to the fetal spine, the presenting part, and thus to the cervix. The term applied to this mechanism is 'fetal axis pressure'. With the membranes intact, the pressure is exerted through the amniotic fluid and distributed equally over the fetus, the cord and the placenta. As labour progresses the internal os dilates, the membranes lose their support, the fetus descends and the presenting part fits well into the lower uterine segment separating the forewaters from the hindwaters.

Even though the pressure intensifies as labour progresses, undue compression is avoided whilst the membranes remain intact. The experience of midwives dealing with labour where intervention is not necessary, is that the membranes normally rupture at the end of the first stage or during the second stage. This is a phenomenon noted in the findings by Schwarz *et al* (1973) in a study relating to late rupture of the membranes. Out of 517 normal labours, 66 per cent of women reached the end of the first stage before the membranes ruptured spontaneously and in 12 per cent the membranes were intact at delivery. Schwartz *et al* reported that the time of highest frequency of spontaneous rupture was full dilation.

It has been known for some time that uterine blood flow is normally affected by contractions reducing oxygen transfer to the fetus (Ramsey 1968) but in normal labour the fetus is unlikely to be compromised. Once the membranes rupture, however, fluid is lost leading to compression of the placenta, umbilical cord and fetus during contractions, leading to increased interruption of the oxygen supply. Brotanek and Hodr (1968) carried out a detailed analysis on 8 pregnant women at term in whom induction of labour was to be carried out. They continuously observed fetal behaviour, uterine activity and uterine blood flow and concluded that amniotomy produces a 'long lasting' reduction of uterine blood flow. They also observed that the introduction of oxytocin at the same time led to a further decrease in blood flow and suggested that administration of oxytocin should be delayed for at least 40 minutes in the interests of the fetus. Donald (1966) stated that the advantage of not rupturing the membranes was an 'intact mother and baby'.

Apart from the reduced likelihood of infection, the other significant benefit of intact membranes is the maintenance of an even hydrostatic pressure to the whole of the fetal surface during labour. Fetal asphyxia is less likely because retraction of the placental site and thus impairment of the utero-placental circulation will not occur. Donald's work was supported by the findings of Schwartz (1961), Althabe (1969) and Caldeyro-Barcia *et al* (1972). Schwartz (1961) found disturbances in the pressure exerted on the fetus, cord and placenta by contractions once the membranes were ruptured. Althabe (1969) confirmed that uneven compression and misalignment of the fetal skull bones after rupture occurred, while Caldeyro-Barcia and colleagues (1974) referred to the occlusion of umbilical vessels leading to marked alterations in fetal heart rate patterns. In presenting his paper at the conference on Modern Perinatal Medicine held in Chicago in 1974, Caldeyro-Barcia commented upon the 'undesirable effects' of early rupture of the membranes on the fetus and recommended 'a critical appraisal' of the practice in the light of the evidence from these studies.Over 1200 women had participated in these studies providing valuable information on the effects of rupture of membranes. In the paper he presented an analysis of the first 1124 pregnancies was given, all of the women were healthy, at term and labour was spontaneous proceeding to normal vaginal delivery. The findings clearly indicated some adverse perinatal effects relating to early amniotomy, as were also suggested by the findings of others (Martell *et al* 1976; Steer *et al* 1976). Small studies by Aladjem (1977) and Stewart *et al* (1982) suggested otherwise however. Sixty-eight women participated in the study carried out by Stewart and colleagues but four were excluded as labour was terminated by caesarean section. In addition, a further 44 would have been excluded from the Caldeyro-Barcia study, so a comparison is difficult to make. The conclusion drawn from this small study was that there were no detrimental effects to the fetus from early amniotomy.

Leaving the membranes intact is considered a disadvantage by many even though there is a distinct lack of evidence supporting the practice of amniotomy. Doctors have claimed that women are pleased with these interventions (Tacchi 1971), though many do not bother to find out their views (RCOG 1977), and still today there are those who believe women should accept whatever is on offer as the professional 'knows best' (Henderson 1984). There are indications, however, that women are becoming more and more concerned with what is happening to them (Oakley 1980) and with what they feel to be the destruction of emotional satisfaction (Raeburn 1981).

The process of birth is regarded as a mechanical process to be controlled with little regard for psychological care (Taylor & Copstick 1985). The overriding of biological norms with medical ones has the undesirable effect of standardising labour and increasing intervention. One intervention may require yet another to negate its effects (Inch 1982). Thus control and domination of the physiological aspects of labour has continued with the stated aim of improving health.

■ Artificial rupture of the membranes (ARM) – the obstetric view

The membranes may be ruptured artificially once the external os starts to dilate. This, it is argued, causes the fetal head to descend allowing the application of greater pressure on the os, creating greater nerve stimulation which leads to stronger contractions and more rapid dilatations. Mitchell (1976) found that there was an increased prostaglandin production when amniotomy was performed, adding support to the extra stimulation view. Others have suggested that a shorter labour reduces the need for operative intervention, but it has been reported (Kitzinger 1975) that shorter labours following amniotomy are more painful, perhaps reflecting the increased production of naturally occurring prostaglandins. Stewart *et al* (1982) commented that shorter labours did not appear to reduce the need for analgesia but failed to detail the analgesia required by the participants in his study.

Once the membranes have been ruptured an electrode can be applied to the fetal head allowing internal electronic monitoring of the fetal heart rate (EMFHR), and the collection of fetal blood for analysis of gases. It is perhaps ironic that the very same person who was the greatest exponent of intact membranes in normal labour, Caldeyro-Barcia, introduced the electronic method for continuous recording of the fetal heart rate. This was in the 1950s but initially it was intended only for use with women who had known risk factors.

Apart from reducing the length of time in labour and making possible the application of a scalp electrode, the other advantage of ARM is that the colour and amount of liquor can be seen and therefore the presence of meconium staining, indicative of fetal distress, detected. There is, however, some controversy about the significance of meconium stained liquor, as discussed by Beazley and Lobb (1983) in their book *Aspects of care in labour*. Some evidence suggests that there is a correlation between meconium stained liquor and *other* signs of fetal distress, but Miller *et al* (1975) reported that 'meconium stained liquor alone does not herald a poor fetal outcome unless other signs of fetal distress are also present', while Meiss and colleagues (1978) found no significance in meconium stained liquor. Earlier, Beard and Campbell (1977) stated that in 40 per cent of stillbirths there was no meconium staining and therefore the *absence* of meconium was not a 'reliable indicator of fetal wellbeing'. Beazley and Lobb conclude:

> The factors which preserve fetal wellbeing and nurture obstetric success need to be further elucidated in order to define safe sensible care of the fetus. Hopefully, future emphasis will be placed on this more positive aspect of care rather than upon an evaluation of the cause of death.

While it may be accepted that the membranes must be ruptured to allow the technique of internal monitoring in order to detect fetal distress during labour, disagreement continues as to whether all 'patients' should be monitored (Edginton *et al* 1975; Baggish & Lee 1976) or whether monitoring should be restricted to those who are in a 'high risk' category (Paul & Hon 1974).

In trying to determine the merits of continuous electronic fetal monitoring versus midwife auscultation with a stethoscope, Macdonald and colleagues (1985) conducted a large randomised controlled trial. Apart from higher intervention rates in the electronically monitored group, the one significant finding between these groups was the greater occurrence of newborn seizures in the intermittently monitored groups as opposed to the electronically monitored group. In an assessment of the babies at one year, however, equal numbers of babies in each group had severe disabilities and the point is made that the relationship between 'intrapartum asphyxia' and long term disability remains controversial. Elsewhere (WHO 1985) the trial is criticised because both groups consisted of 'altered women and babies':

> It was later found that this difference between the two groups applied only to those labours that had been artificially induced.
>
> This may be an instance of one intervention necessitating another. Furthermore what is the normal incidence of newborn seizures?
>
> All the women in this hospital are subjected to active management of labour, which means that both groups experienced a specific obstetric approach beyond the monitoring in question. The findings still depend on the context. Until the incidence of seizures in infants having a 'non-medicalized' birth is known, little can be said about this result beyond the fact that women giving birth under similar conditions have infants altered in these particular ways. (Page 85).

The conclusion of those conducting the study is that there is little justification for the use of electronic fetal heart monitoring without facilities to assess fetal acid base status. Others have questioned the value of internal EMFHR monitoring as many professionals are not able to interpret the recordings adequately. In an editorial, Simkin (1987) highlights the results of six trials concerning electronic fetal monitoring and states:

> One might expect that the lack of evidence of clear benefit would influence clinicians and hospital administrators to rely less on EFM than they now do. Alternatively, if they are persuaded of the benefit of EFM's association with a reduction in neonatal seizures, one might expect that internal EFM with fetal scalp blood sampling would become the standard of care. In fact, neither of these choices has been adopted by most hospitals. Routine policies on the use of EFM vary.

Fetal monitoring continues to stimulate debate about risks, effectiveness and costs, in terms of both wellbeing and finance.

■ Artificial rupture of the membranes – how valuable is it?

The arguments put forward in favour of ARM have been discussed above. The results of an NCT survey reported by Kitzinger (1975), however, considered that the length of labour was perhaps less crucial than the degree and quality of emotional support. One might argue that electronic fetal monitoring is essential in modern childbirth management, an expectation of many mothers and a security for professionals, even though the evidence suggests that it is of limited value especially in 'low risk' cases. Many argue, however, that there is no such thing as low risk labour and that the detection of anoxia is imperative for a good perinatal outcome, although the method of detection is controversial. Klein *et al* (1983) highlight the fact that the style of management is, and needs to be, different in 'low' and 'high' risk cases otherwise there is the tendency to intervene unnecessarily treating everyone as 'high risk'. They conclude that the traditional role of midwives is justifiable in the management of 'low risk' women.

After a consideration of *all* the evidence available the conclusions highlighted in the WHO (1985) report *Having a baby in Europe* was that, 'early rupture of the membranes as a routine process is not scientifically justified'. Who then should make the decision regarding this procedure? Should it be left to the obstetrician or the midwife? Does the 'professional know best?' What are the views of those using the maternity services? How do they feel?

■ Artificial rupture of the membranes – the 'consumer' view

Recognition of the need for close study of the woman's point of view is nothing new (Royal Commission on Population, 1949). Sometimes, however, in the paraphernalia surrounding the circumstances of childbirth, many feel that they have no rights and that they are not given the information they need to participate in decisions about their own bodies. In many instances, they are not consulted but just told (Kirkham 1983) what has been decided and is going to be done. With the reduction in mortality rates and improved socioeconomic circumstances, mothers and babies are healthier and the fear of death is diminished. Many women now feel, therefore, that having a baby is a normal physiological process to be enjoyed and not a medical disorder to be endured. The father's right to be present and to give active support to his partner in the labour ward has altered the sociodynamics of the situation, in that there is now a third party present whose needs have to be considered.

No longer are the majority of women ignorant, passive and compliant. They are informed, many are articulate, and all encouraged by self help or pressure groups to state their own wishes. The conclusions of the BBC series 'That's Life' in 1981 (6000 surveyed) were that many women were demanding the right to be treated as individuals, wishing to be consulted and make decisions about what happens to them.

The opening words to the Maternity Services Advisory Committee's (1984) second report on intrapartum care states:

> Staff must recognise that mothers are healthy women for whom labour and birth are important physiological and emotional events. A mother is not necessarily 'a patient' and should not normally be referred to as such.

The report was given support by the DHSS which recognised that there was 'undoubted justification' for the dissatisfactions with services expressed, attributing this to increased technology. Dissatisfaction also comes from some who complain of too little intervention, too few tests and screening procedures and complications being missed. The central theme of the report is the need for consultation, discussion and agreement with each mother, and an individual plan for her care during labour and childbirth. Some women prefer to cede control to the experts. In 1977, Riley asked the question 'What do women want?' The answer appeared to be that this varies; in the management of labour women may want different things but on 'a common foundation of humane treatment'.

Very little research has been undertaken seeking the views of mothers with regard to rupture of the membranes. Perhaps for the majority it is considered a necessary intervention before the birth itself. When mothers were asked for their views regarding discussion before the midwife ruptures the membranes, Henderson (1984) found that the majority did not think it necessary and some indicated that as the professional 'she knew best'. See Table 3.1 for a summary of the comments received from those participating. The study was conducted in a health authority serving a multiracial, socially deprived group of mothers and, although small (28 women participated), probably reflects the views of a larger number of women.

The following extracts are taken from interviews with women in labour who thought that the midwife should discuss and tell more. The midwife concerned was not present when the mothers were interviewed.

Gravida 1, West Indian, aged 21:
> The midwife mentioned about 'breaking the waters' and putting the monitor on the baby's head. I minded the waters being broken... I didn't really want them broken but it was too late to say anything. I would have liked more discussion about the clip on the baby's head. I was just told it would be put on.

Table 3.1   What women said in relation to rupture of membranes

Midwife knows best	4
Do not think needs discussion	13
Midwife did discuss	6
Midwife should discuss/tell more	3
No replies	2

Gravida 6, white caucasian, aged 37

The midwife told me, I wanted to know but then I didn't want to know everything she was doing... Really you've no choice in the matter. If I refused it would take longer, perhaps harm the baby, but you should be asked.

Gravida 2, white caucasian, aged 22

The midwife didn't ask me, she just told me she was going to break them. I suppose I didn't mind. It must be alright if they think so. She should have asked though and explained more about the clip on the baby's head.

Perhaps this is what many women feel but fail to express verbally to the midwife. The majority of women did not think there should be discussion regarding rupture of the membranes and quite often said that they were happy for the midwife to go ahead, implying that 'she knew best'. Four specifically said this. Other comments within this group were:

– It'll help the contractions
– Have to be broken before baby comes
– Labour doesn't take as long
– It happens more quickly

Two women who were happy for the midwife to carry on 'at the time' were quite advanced in labour and were interviewed afterwards. Both commented on the fetal scalp electrode. In fact it was this procedure that one consultant felt should generate discussion and that all women should be consulted prior to it's application. Perhaps different comments would have been forthcoming had the women been interviewed after delivery when they were physically less dependent upon their attendants and would therefore have felt freer to comment.

Table 3.2 summarises the answers of the midwives when asked the

Table 3.2   Midwives' replies to 'Why didn't you discuss your decision to rupture membranes?'

Mother did not ask questions	8
Never discuss	6
She knew all about it (usually had it done before)	4
Did discuss	2
Didn't think of it	2
Doctor told me to do it	2
No time, going to be busy	1
Lack of understanding	1
Mother said 'water' already gone	1
Discussed previously	1

question, 'Why didn't you think it appropriate to discuss your decision to rupture the membranes with this woman?' If one compares these answers with answers received to the question, 'Would you *ever* discuss whether to rupture the membranes or not with the mother?', 19 stated that they would only do so if the mother asked questions. The midwife looking after one woman said she did not discuss the decision because there were no questions asked, and went on to say, 'It depends who the mother is and her under-standing ... if she wants to know ... people go along with what you do.' She would discuss if asked questions.

This assumes that if the woman does want to know she will ask questions, but this is not always the case. Macintyre (1982) states that this is an assumption common where working class women are concerned. Some women feel unable to ask questions because of their unfamiliarity with the environment and their dependence during labour. Nine said they would never discuss. The majority might have felt obliged to say yes. Two midwives did answer that it hadn't crossed their minds to discuss their decision with the client before participating in the survey. Midwives' re-plies to the question 'What factors would you take into consideration when deciding whether or not to discuss the intervention?' are set out in Table 3.3.

Since all of the women included in the study could understand English, some were in early labour, and some did ask questions, it could have been expected that discussion would have occurred. Of the nine midwives who said they would not discuss their decision, 6 made the comment that if the

Table 3.3   Factors taken into consideration by midwives determining discussion

Factors	No of midwives
Only if asks questions	8
Understanding of English	6
Stage of labour (early)	4
Parity (if first)	1
TOTAL	19

woman refused to have their membranes ruptured, they would go on to discuss the reasons why the procedure should be carried out.

Very little discussion and no consultation with the women took place when the decision to rupture the membranes was made. What happens in the majority of instances is illustrated in the following comments typical of many made by the midwives:

> You come to mother and say, 'I'm just going to examine you and break the waters', and she usually accepts.

This passive acceptance was borne out by the author's observations, although not all of the women included in the survey were entirely happy with the situation. Many appeared to be more resigned to the fact that the membranes have to rupture before the baby is born and that labour in their experience was usually quicker once the 'waters' had broken. The midwives seemed to assume that no questions implied agreement and therefore saw no need for discussion. One midwife told the mother she was going to 'break the waters' asking 'is that all right?' The mother said 'I have no choice'. The midwife said 'yes you have' – and carried on with the procedure. If the mothers had been assertive in challenging the midwife then this might have made a difference both in obtaining consent to the actual procedure and/or in influencing the decision.

The findings of this small descriptive study were that although the midwives were good at explaining what they were going to do, there was:

- No discussion before rupturing the membranes (consent was obtained in two instances out of 22 observed cases);

- A misconception on the part of the midwives that they were using their own judgement while in fact they were unwittingly following a routine in part due to medical pressure;

- There was a passive acceptance by the women involved which probably served to reinforce the practices.

The view that the professional 'knows best' still applies for the majority who are resigned to accepting what the system has to offer. It seems that only a minority feel able to challenge. Other studies, however, have commented on the impact that the womens' movement has had in raising awareness and expectations (Jacoby 1987) and helping women to be more positive in making their views known. In Jacoby's retrospective study, 72 per cent of mothers had hoped not to have artificial rupture of membranes but the procedure was carried out in over half of the cases. The mothers' initial wishes were not met and they fell within the group dissatisfied with the management of labour. Unfortunately there was insufficient information to form any conclusions relating to frequency of depression associated with artificial rupture of membranes. It was stated that there is a relationship between procedures and depression postnatally, but the data collected was insufficient for any real conclusions. The point was made, however, that women's views about procedures need to be taken into account.

Perhaps the procedures themselves are of less concern than the quality of communication. McIntosh (1988) was encouraged that his findings showed progress in the level of communication compared with the previous studies he looked at, but he claimed that there still was room for improvement.

The largest ever survey (NCT 1989) seeking mothers' views on rupture of the membranes in labour has been published recently. The majority of the 3000 women who responded didn't want the procedure performed, partly because labour became more painful and partly because they considered that it would interfere with the normal physiological process. The data is rich with first hand accounts of mothers' experiences and of the reactions of midwives to those requesting 'intact' membranes. It also highlights the fact that those delivering in a hospital setting, either GP or consultant unit or within a domino scheme, were more likely to have artificial rupture of membranes.

Some would argue that these women are the articulate few unrepresentative of the population. One must not forget, however, that they represent a proportion of the population using the services and we must be sensitive to the needs of *all* women, helping them to identify their needs and anxieties, and assisting them to realise their wishes where possible. Those who wish to be involved should be encouraged to participate in decisions, those who prefer to leave midwives and obstetricians to take the decisions regarding care need to be kept informed of what is happening. Midwives are in a unique position, they can act as advocates and to a larger extent determine the quality of communication and social climate in the labour ward. It is they who can make the difference between an experience which is a unique and special occasion or one that is quite otherwise.

■ Recommendations for clinical practice in the light of currently available evidence

1. Early rupture of the membranes as routine practice is not scientifically justified.

2. Research suggests that where there is a significant risk to fetal wellbeing, then artificial rupture of the membranes is necessary to facilitate the application of a fetal scalp electrode so that internal continuous electronic fetal monitoring can be initiated. In low risk cases the disadvantages of artificial rupture of the membranes (such as a more painful labour) may outweigh the advantages. Health authority policies, both formal and informal, should be reviewed in the light of this.

3. Where internal fetal monitoring is required, research suggests that fetal blood sampling should also be performed.

4. Mothers should be consulted in the decision making process regarding artificial rupture of the membranes. Those wishing to be involved should be encouraged to participate in the decision; those wishing to leave the decision to the professionals should be kept informed about what is happening and the reasons for the decision should be explained.

5. Antenatal teaching should include discussion of all aspects of the procedure and should foster critical awareness in clients.

6. The education of midwives relating to the practice of artificial rupture of the membranes should include a study of available research thus allowing them to make informed decisions rather than following routine practice.

7. The communication surrounding artificial rupture of the membranes is as important as the procedure itself.

■ Practice check

- Do you provide discussion regarding the advantages and disadvantages of artificial rupture of the membranes in antenatal education and preparation classes?

- Do you encourage mothers and their partners to participate in the decision regarding artificial rupture of the membranes during labour?

- How well do you communicate with mothers on all aspects of their care during pregnancy, labour and the puerperium?

- Do you obtain consent from the mother for all the procedures that you perform?

- Does your health authority have an informal or formal policy relating to artificial rupture of the membranes and when it should be performed during labour? Does this need to be reviewed in the light of current research?

- Have midwives and doctors in your own unit developed routines in communicating with mothers, or in the procedures they perform? If so, should these routines provide a point of discussion and regular review at unit meetings?

- Have you a mechanism within your unit for appraising the views and expectations of mothers and their partners concerning all aspects of pregnancy, labour and the puerperium? If not should you consider the development and implementation of such a mechanism?

■ References

Aladjem S, Miller T 1977 Effects of spontaneous and artificial membrane rupture in labour upon fetal heart rate. British Journal of Obstetrics and Gynaecology 84: 44–7

Althabe O 1969 Influence of the rupture of membranes on compression of the fetal head during labour. In Caldeyro-Barcia R (ed) Perinatal factors affecting human development. Pan American Health Organisation, Washington DC

Baggish M, Lee W 1976 The effect of unselected intrapartum fetal monitoring. Obstetrics and Gynaecology 47: 516

Beard R, Campbell S (eds) 1977 Current status of fetal heart rate monitoring and ultrasound in obstetrics. RCOG, London

Beazley J, Lobb M 1983 Aspects of care in labour: 80. Churchill Livingstone, Edinburgh

Brotanek V, Hodr J 1968 Fetal distress after artificial rupture of the membranes. American Journal of Obstetrics and Gynecology 101: 542

Caldeyro-Barcia R, Schwartz R L, Athlabe O 1972 Effects of rupture of the membranes on fetal heart rate pattern. International Journal of Gynaecology and Obstetrics 10: 169

Caldeyro-Barcia R, Schwartz R, Belizau R *et al* 1974 Adverse perinatal effects of early amniotomy during labour. In Gluck L (ed) Modern perinatal medicine. Year Book Medical Publishers, Chicago

Chalmers I, Richards M 1977 Intervention and causal inference in obstetric practice. In Benefits and hazards of the new obstetrics. Heinemann, London

Comaroff J 1977 Conflicting paradigms of pregnancy. In Davis A, Horobin G (eds) Medical Encounters. Croom Helm, London

Donald I 1966 Practical obstetric problems. Lloyd Luke, London

Edginton P T, Sibanda J, Beard R W 1975 Influence on clinical practice of routine intrapartum monitoring. British Medical Journal 3: 341–43

Henderson, C 1984 Influences and interactions surrounding the decision to rupture the membranes by the midwife. Unpublished MA dissertation, University of Warwick

Inch S 1982 Birthright: a parents' guide to modern childbirth. Hutchinson, London

Jacoby A 1987 Womens' preferences for and satisfaction with current procedures in childbirth – Findings from a national study. Midwifery 3: 117–24

Kirkham M 1983 Admission in labour: teaching the patient to be patient. Midwives Chronicle 96(2): 44–5

Kitzinger S 1975 Some mothers' experience of induced labour. National Childbirth Trust, London

Kitzinger S 1988 The midwife challenge. Pandora Press, London

Klein M, Lloyd I, Redman C et al 1983 A comparison of low risk pregnant women booked for delivery in two systems of care: shared care (consultant) and integrated general practice unit. British Journal of Obstetrics and Gynaecology 90: 123–28

Macdonald D, Grant A, Sheridan-Pereira M et al 1985 The Dublin randomised controlled trial of intrapartum fetal heart rate monitoring. American Journal of Obstetrics and Gynecology 138: 524–39

Macintyre S 1982 Communications between pregnant women and their medical and midwifery attendants. Midwives Chronicle 95: 387–94

Martell M, Belizau J M, Niets F, Schwartz R 1976 Blood acid–base balance at birth in neonates from labours with early and late rupture of membranes. Journal of Paediatrics 89: 963–67

Maternity Services Advisory Committee 1984 Maternity care in action, part II: Care during childbirth (intrapartum care). HMSO, London

McIntosh J 1988 Women's views of communication during labour and delivery. Midwifery 4: 166–70

Meiss P J, Hall N, Marshall J R 1978 Meconium passage: a new classification for risk assessment in labor. American Journal of Obstetrics and Gynecology 131: 509–13

Miller S C, Sacks D A, Yeh S et al 1975 Significance of meconium during labor. American Journal of Obstetrics and Gynecology 122: 573

Mitchell M D, Flint A P F, Bibby J et al 1976 Rapid increases in plasma prostaglandin concentrations after vaginal examination and amniotomy. British Medical Journal 3: 1183–85

National Childbirth Trust 1989 Rupture of the membranes in labour: women's views. NCT, London

Oakley A 1980 Women confined. Robertson, London

Paul R H, Hon E H 1974 Clinical fetal monitoring vs effect on perinatal outcome. American Journal of Obstetrics and Gynecology 118: 529–32

Raeburn J 1981 Hospital delivery. British Journal of Hospital Medicine 282: 822

Ramsey E M 1968 Uteroplacental circulation during labour. Clinical Obstetrics and Gynaecology II: 78

Riley E M D 1977 What do women want? the question of choice in the conduct of labour. In Chalmers I, Richards M (eds) Benefits and hazards of the new obstetrics. Heinemann, London

Royal College of Obstetricians and Gynaecologists 1977 Current Status of fetal heart rate monitoring and ultrasound in obstetrics. RCOG, London

Royal Commission on Population 1949 Command paper CMD 7695. HMSO, London

Schwartz P 1961 Birth injury of the newborn. Hafner New York

Schwartz R, Belizou J M, Nieto F, Tenzer S M 1973 Fetal heart rate patterns in labours with intact and with ruptured membranes. Journal of Perinatal Medicine I: 153

Simkin P 1987 Is anyone listening? The lack of clinical impact of randomised controlled trials of electronic fetal monitoring. Birth 13(4): 219–20

Steer P J, Little D J, Lewis N L *et al* 1976 Effect of membrane rupture on fetal heart rate in induced labour. British Journal of Obstetrics and Gynaecology 83: 544–49

Stewart P, Kennedy J H, Calder A A 1982 Spontaneous labour: when should the membranes be ruptured? British Journal of Obstetrics and Gynaecology 89: 39

Tacchi D 1971 Towards easier childbirth. Lancet ii: 1134–36

Taylor K, Copstick S 1985 Psychological care in labour. Nursing Mirror 161(4): 42–3

World Health Organisation 1985 Having a baby in Europe. Public Health in Europe 26. WHO, Geneva

■ Suggested further reading

Kirkham M 1989 Midwives and information giving in labour. In Robinson S, Thomson A (eds) Midwives, research and childbirth. Chapman and Hall, London

Maternity Services Advisory Committee 1984 'Maternity Care in Action' Part II. Care during childbirth (intrapartum care). HMSO, London. Contains action checklists at the end of each chapter concerning policies and practices

MIDIRS packs 1986 (No 3); 1987 (No 5) – useful extracts from published research worldwide, reports and information on all aspects of childbirth. They also have a database and will, for a small charge, mount a literature search

National Childbirth Trust 1989 Rupture of the membranes in labour: women's views. NCT, London

Chapter 4

Nutrition and hydration in labour

Judith Grant

Most textbooks of midwifery or obstetric practice make only cursory reference to nutrition and hydration in labour. Many make unsubstantiated statements to the effect that women in active labour should be allowed only sips of water or ice to suck, one being left to assume that the main reason is to minimise the risk of acid aspiration should a general anaesthetic be required. (Pearce 1987; Power 1987.)

The problem with this approach is that labour is hard, sustained work. Muscles only store sufficient glycogen for short bursts of energy production and therefore require a continuous supply of glycogen (Katch & McArdle 1983), either from limited liver stores or from the diet. A normal labour can last in excess of 12 hours and if the woman is not provided with an energy source she will suffer the effects of hunger, both physically and psychologically. The result will be muscle fatigue, prolonged labour and a lowered pain threshold.

Many in the medical profession are confident that they can provide the energy required by intravenous infusion. Several writers on both sides of the Atlantic, however, question such blanket policies. Although research in this area has been limited, this chapter will discuss the arguments for and against oral nutrition and hydration, together with the problems caused by intravenous infusion.

■ **It is assumed that you are already aware of the following:**

● The physiology of muscle action;

● The physiology of labour with special reference to the gastro-intestinal system;

- The reasons why general anaesthesia may be required during labour;
- The risks of general anaesthesia during labour.

■ Critical appraisal of the literature

There appear to be two very definite schools of thought regarding nutrition in labour. One group, mainly comprised of obstetric anaesthetists, wish all labouring clients to be treated as pre-surgery patients whose stomachs are kept empty for fear of aspiration of stomach acid during induction or recovery from general anaesthesia. The other group, mainly midwives and the women themselves, prefer to view labour as a normal event more akin to work or sport than illness.

□ The case for oral nutrition during labour

Very little appears to have been published about allowing oral nutrition during labour, although policies vary widely within different hospitals. In most units a 'nil by mouth' ruling applies for clients in labour (Macleod 1987) even though 75 per cent of clients in England and Wales are delivered with the midwife as the most senior person in attendance (Robinson *et al* 1983), having had no need for a general anaesthetic.

Ludka (1987) reported that in New York's North Central Bronx Hospital clients in labour were allowed to eat lightly and drink as they pleased, except for a six month period between July 1983 and January 1984. During this time the use of chemicals to stimulate labour increased fivefold, delivery by instruments increased by 35 per cent and caesarean section by 38 per cent, the need for neonatal intensive care rose by 69 per cent and the only case of maternal aspiration for ten years occurred during this period in a client who had taken nil by mouth for 36 hours. As a result of the adverse effects upon maternal and fetal outcome when the clients were starved, this hospital returned to its previous policy of allowing more liberal oral nutrition during labour, although Ludka does not specify what is meant by a light diet.

In her experience of caring for clients who have chosen to aim for natural labour (that is labour where no pain relieving drugs are taken and there is no intervention), Milner (1986) advocates encouraging the clients to eat a light meal or take hot drinks of tea or water with honey. The clients should also be encouraged to drink large amounts of cold water. With this regimen she found surprisingly few intravenous infusions were required for ketosis.

In the contrasting culture of Haryana, North India, a survey of home deliveries (Walia 1986) showed the women were mainly cared for by the female members of their families or traditional birth attendants. The traditional care of the labouring women resulted in 52 per cent of women taking milk, 44 per cent dried fruits and condiments such as ginger and 25 per cent tea. The majority of these women (92.8 per cent) had no problems during labour and 91.2 per cent of the newborn were also well.

Hazle (1986) would liken the labouring client to an endurance athlete such as a marathon runner. The carbohydrate loading pre-event meal and frequent intake of diluted glucose-electrolyte solution during the event has been shown to improve an athlete's performance (Lancet 1987). The result of undertaking such an endurance event, without nutrition and fluid replacement, leads to the build-up of toxic metabolites which can activate the vomiting centre and cause nausea and vomiting with extreme muscle fatigue. The same can be seen in labouring women who are denied oral intake.

Broach and Newtown (1988) suggest the psychological effect of prohibiting food has been overlooked in the literature. They maintain that meals, and even tea, coffee or soft drinks have a mood elevating effect on many clients. They report a study by Simkin (1986) which found that 50 per cent of those whose oral intake was restricted found this 'stressful' or 'most stressful'. Prohibiting food will also have physiological effects. Guyton (1986) states:

> In a person who has not had food for many hours, the stomach undergoes intense rhythmic contractions... These cause a tight or gnawing feeling in the pit of the stomach and sometimes actually cause pain. The hungry person becomes more tense and restless than usual. (Page 863)

In other words, without food the woman in labour will begin to feel ill and apprehensive. These induced stress factors can lead to an increased level of circulating catecholamines. The result may be increased arterial pressure, increased blood flow to active muscle with corresponding decrease to organs not needed for rapid activity. Raised catecholamine levels may also increase cellular metabolism and the demand for glucose, and will affect muscle strength, mental activity and the rate of blood coagulation (Guyton 1986: 695). Is it any wonder then that when obstetricians of the North Central Bronx Hospital ceased to allow clients light nourishment and oral fluids throughout labour they found such a change in outcome both for the women and for the newborn?

□ Ketonuria in labour

Whether the client is allowed to take oral nourishment or not, the uterus in labour will continue to contract and demand an energy supply. The non-pregnant body only stores a few hundred grammes of carbohydrate, sufficient to supply the energy requirements for body function for approximately 12 hours (Guyton 1986: 866). Metzger *et al* (1982) showed that pregnant women who are starved during the third trimester rapidly became hypoglycaemic and this phenomenon will be accentuated in labour (Dumoulin & Foulkes 1984). The body's response to this shortage of glucose will be to metabolise fat into free fatty acids which are progressively broken down in the liver to produce acetyl-coenzyme-A. Pairs of these molecules combine to form aceto-acetic acid and three hydroxybutyric acid (ketone bodies). These ketone bodies travel to the cells where they are converted back to acetyl-coenzyme-A and enter the Kreb's cycle taking place within the mitochondria of the muscle cells, to form energy (Katch & McArdle 1983). Cells will not, however, be able to cope immediately with the rise in ketone bodies and some will be excreted as ketonuria (Guyton 1986: 823). Thus ketone bodies *per se* are not toxic substances and they will appear in maternal urine before hyperketonaemia and subsequent acidosis are present (Chez & Curcio 1987). Ketonuria is also seen in athletes, particularly *after* endurance events. Because ketonuria occurs *during* labour, Paterson *et al* (1967) maintain that this cannot be compared with that occurring in sportsmen; however, the marathon runner does not stop running for the 2–4 hours of his event, whereas the contracting uterus does not normally sustain a contraction for longer than a minute nor contract more frequently than once every three minutes for most of the labour. Paterson and colleagues (1967) argued that the physical exertion was unlikely to be the cause of ketonuria because ketone levels were found to be higher in women who had been starved for 12 hours prior to elective caesarean section than women who had laboured. This ties in with the previously mentioned work of Metzger *et al* (1982). Paterson *et al* found no change in maternal or fetal acid-base status, nor reduced maternal glucose when ketonuria was present and yet they still considered it necessary to remove the ketones by intravenous glucose infusion. A further interesting point from this article was that the level of ketones found in cord blood was lower than in the maternal plasma and the authors' suggest that the placenta is also able to convert ketones efficiently into energy. Where the placenta was compromised however (as in the case of severe pre-eclampsia) the cord ketones were higher than in maternal plasma and there is a fear that this could lead to fetal brain damage.

From the literature reviewed, it would seem that mild ketonuria is a normal physiological occurrence. The body is only able to store limited amounts of glycogen but can store large amounts of fat. The pregnant woman's fat stores markedly increase and the utilisation of this fat will result in less expendable fuels, such as glucose, being saved for the growth and well being of the fetus (Metzger *et al* 1982). Interference in this physiological adjustment by giving intravenous glucose may, however, cause more problems than it is supposed to prevent.

■ Intravenous fluid administration during labour

For a long time obstetricians believed that ketonuria in labour interfered with uterine action and they therefore treated the clients vigorously with intravenous fluids (Dumoulin & Foulkes 1984). From the literature it would appear that the routine use of intravenous fluids in labour was much more common in America than in Britain. Authors on both sides of the Atlantic, however, are now questioning their use and agree (Macleod 1987; Douglas 1988) that the three main reasons for prescribing intravenous fluids are:

- For correction of Ketoacidosis and dehydration;

- As a vehicle for the administration of drugs such as oxytocin;

- During establishment and maintenance of epidural anaesthesia.

These indications will now be discussed.

□ Correction of ketoacidosis and dehydration

Tarnow-Mordi *et al* (1981) found no data on the effect of ketosis on uterine action nor on the value of glucose infusion in the treatment of mild ketosis. It has, however, been shown that where more than 25 g Dextrose is given intravenously (one litre of Dextrose 5 per cent in water will contain 50 g of Dextrose), maternal blood glucose will rise and there will be a corresponding rise in umbilical arterial insulin and lactate with a lowering of pH (Kenepp *et al* 1982). This will result in the newborn becoming hypoglycaemic within two hours of birth due to its removal from the hyperglycaemic conditions where it had been stimulated to produce its own insulin. There was also evidence that these infants developed a level of jaundice greater than those whose mothers had been given less than 25 g of Dextrose. As a result of this, Kenepp and colleagues suggested that Dextrose infusion should be limited to 6 g/hour for those undergoing elective caesarean section. Evans *et al* (1986) advocate an infusion rate of 10 g/hour of Dextrose for clients undergoing induced labour, in order to prevent severe ketosis (Mendiola *et al* 1982).

Hazle (1986) points out that ketonuria is often cited as being indicative that the labouring client is dehydrated, thus again apparently justifying the use of intravenous fluids. Before intravenous fluids are considered for the correction of dehydration, it is important to have an understanding of the fluid balance during labour. Macleod (1987) describes water distribution by dividing total body water into extracellular and intracellular compartments (see Fig. 4.1). Lind (1983) highlights the difficulties of using these divisions in terms of accuracy, but for descriptive purposes they are useful when considering the changes which occur in pregnancy. The total body fluid of the pregnant woman increases by 6 to 10 litres, depending on the degree of

Figure 4.1 Water distribution in the adult

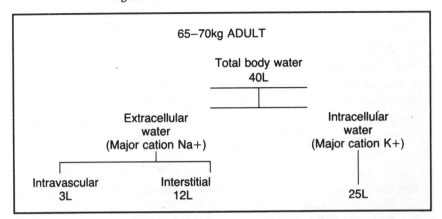

Source: K. G. Macleod, 'Analgesia and Nutrition and the Mother's Choice in Labour' *Midwife, Health Visitor and Community Nurse* vol. 23 No. 9 September 1987 p. 409 Newbourne Publishers Ltd.

oedema present. Between 3 and 6 litres of this will be in the extracellular compartment.

During pregnancy plasma osmolality is reduced by about 10 mosmol/ kg. In the non-pregnant state, a similar reduction in plasma osmolality would occur after drinking one litre of water. This would result in suppression of antidiuretic hormone and water diuresis returning osmolality to normal within two hours. During the first and second trimesters of pregnancy, the resulting reduction in osmolality from drinking one litre of water would be corrected to the new lower level by diuresis in the same way but more quickly. In the third trimester, however, although osmolality is maintained, urine volume does not increase in response to drinking the water, therefore the extra water must leave the intravascular compartment for the extravascular space (Lind 1983). From here it is excreted slowly – which is perhaps the reason for increased nocturia. The significance of this is that any increased fluid load is not excreted promptly. During labour excretion of excess water is further delayed by an increased level of plasma antidiuretic hormone, possibly caused by the rise in endogenous catecholamines produced in response to pain or fear (Tarnow-Mordi *et al* 1981). Tarnow-Mordi and colleagues also found evidence to suggest that oxytocin has an antidiuretic effect.

Thus Lind (1983), Macleod (1987) and Tarnow-Mordi *et al* (1981) agree that since the client entering labour is fairly 'waterlogged' she is very unlikely to become dehydrated under normal circumstances. Where it is deemed necessary to give intravenous fluids because the client is being given nil orally, labour is prolonged or there is evidence of dehydration and moderate ketosis, then it is important that the fluid balance is carefully

Figure 4.2   Distribution of commonly available fluids after administration

Fluid	Distribution
1L 5% Dextrose	Total body water
1L Dextrose/saline (30 mmolNa+)	Total body water
1L Normal saline (150 mmolNa+)	Extracellular comp
1L Hartmann's solution (131 mmolNa+)	Extracellular comp
1L Dextrose 70 ⎫ Colloid 1L Haemacel ⎭	Intravascular comp Intravascular comp
	Appropriate solution
For: Maintenance	Dextrose/saline
Extracellular loss	Hartmann's solution
Intravenous replacement	Colloid or blood

Source: K. G. Macleod, 'Analgesia and Nutrition and Mother's Choice in Labour' *Midwife, Health Visitor and Community Nurse* vol. 23 No. 9 September 1987 p. 410 Newbourne Publishers Ltd.

controlled. Macleod (1987) recommends 1.0 to 1.5ml/kg/hour, which will be sufficient to replace normal losses. It is important that this fluid contains sodium and is iso-osmotic because if a fluid is given which enters the intracellular compartment (see Fig. 4.2) both client and fetus may suffer water intoxication and hyponatraemia which can prove fatal to the client, and have serious effects on the newborn (Tarnow-Mordi *et al* 1981).

□   Administration of intravenous drugs

The most common drug given intravenously is oxytocin to augment or induce labour. The vehicle for administration of oxytocin is usually 5 per cent Dextrose and Macleod (1987) suggests that this can result in as much as 3 litres being administered in 24 hours, sufficient to cause symptoms of water intoxication in both client and newborn. It is therefore important that the infusion is given in as concentrated a form as is safely possible, that accurate infusion pumps are available for use and that fluid balance records are accurately maintained.

□   Epidural anaesthesia

Lind (1983) is fairly scathing about the use of large volumes of fluid to compensate for the vasodilation and resulting hypotension caused by epidural anaesthesia. If this sudden hypotension is unaccompanied by a raised cardiac output, however, it can predispose to aorta-caval compression and a reduced blood supply to the placenta and must therefore be counteracted (Macleod 1987). This said, it is very important that an appropriate intravenous fluid is used (see Fig. 4.2). The fluid must contain sodium and be iso-osmotic, so that it does not enter the intracellular compartment as discussed previously. For the purpose of raising blood pressure, colloid solutions would at first glance appear to be the most appropriate; however, there is a possibility of anaphylactoid reaction and the risk of circulatory overload with the contraction of the circulatory system after delivery. Hartmann's solution or normal saline are both suitable but these solutions will enter the extravascular compartment and may therefore increase the problem of oedema. Where there is evidence of hypotension persisting, it is physiologically more sound to give a vaso-pressor drug like ephedrine rather than large volumes of fluid (Macleod 1987).

■ Fasting during labour

Pritchard *et al* (1985) and Beazley (1986) categorically state that women in established labour should not be allowed food or oral fluids. Beazley's argument is that 'Normal labour can only be diagnosed in retrospect' and 'on admission to hospital patients in suspected labour should be treated as though at sometime during the next 12 hours a caesarean section will be necessary'. The 'Confidential enquiries into maternal deaths for England and Wales' (DHSS 1989) indicate that women continue to die each year as a direct result of anaesthesia, the two main causes being failure to intubate and Mendelson's syndrome. No one would disagree with Douglas (1988) when she states that pulmonary aspiration is a devastating event exacting a heavy toll from the client, her family and all involved in her care if she survives or dies, but the question still remains as to how long it is necessary or wise to starve a client. What will be the long term effect of such starvation, particularly if it is during the high energy demanding muscular activity of labour? In 1977 Hill *et al* studied the nutritional status of 105 post-operative patients and found evidence of protein-calorie malnutrition, anaemia and depleted vitamin stores in almost 50 per cent of cases. One wonders if clients who undergo caesarean section after a long labour, where only glucose and electrolytes have been given intravenously, are similarly compromised.

Many researchers into preoperative fasting have shown that there is little benefit in starving patients prior to general anaesthesia for longer than four hours (Thomas 1987). It is generally believed however that, due to the action of progesterone, stomach emptying is slower in the latter part of pregnancy and even more so during labour. Two quite different studies

(Holdsworth 1978; Nimmo *et al* 1975) showed that clients in labour have significantly reduced gastric emptying only if they have received narcotics. In contrast, Lewis and Crawford's (1987) study of 40 women prior to elective caesarean section showed that women starved overnight had only half the stomach contents of those given tea and toast or just tea 2.6 to 3.6 hours prior to anaesthetic.

Increased volume of stomach contents is not the only problem faced by obstetric anaesthetists. Due to progesterone and the upward displacement of the stomach by the gravid uterus, the cardiac sphincter is less efficient and allows passive leak of stomach contents into the pharynx when conscious-ness is lost during general anaesthesia. Added to this, the oedema often present in late pregnancy will make intubation more difficult. But are these genuine reasons for starving all women? Macleod (1987) writes, 'Dietary restrictions and antacid regimens have not led to the expected reduction in anaesthetic mortality in the last 20 years and ... this fall can only be achieved by ... provision of experienced and committed anaesthetic help pre-, intra- and post-operatively.'

From these discussions, then it would seem that a blanket policy denying oral nourishment in labour is inappropriate for many women. Indeed, the effects of denying oral intake may cause more problems than the policy solves and may even deny the client the normal delivery she has the potential to achieve. It should be possible to demonstrate that there is a group of clients who can accurately be identified as low risk in terms of their need for general anaesthesia. Having shown this, it could be ethically possible to prove or disprove the hypothesis that allowing clients in labour to eat a light diet when hungry and drink when thirsty will aid progress of their labour, reduce the need for pain relieving drugs and give the women a better opportunity to enjoy their labour.

■ Recommendations for clinical practice in the light of currently available evidence

1. Where it is considered that the client in labour has no risk factors for requiring instrumental delivery or general anaesthesia, she should be allowed to eat a light diet and drink as she requires. A light diet should contain foods which are easily absorbed by the stomach. It will therefore be very low in fats and roughage and only small amounts should be eaten at one time.

2. The presence of small amounts of ketones in the urine can be interpreted as being a normal physiological occurrence.

3. When narcotics are given for pain relief, oral intake of food should cease and water intake be reduced to sips only.

4. When intravenous fluids are administered, an accurate fluid balance record must be maintained. The administration rate should not exceed 1.5ml/kg/hour, nor should the fluid contain more than 10g of Dextrose per hour. Iso-osmotic fluids such as Dextrose/saline or Hartmann's solution should be used.

■ Practice check

● How effective is your assessment of clients in terms of their likely requirement of instrumental delivery or general anaesthesia?

● Do you know how your clients feel about prohibition of food or free fluids during labour?

● Do you know how your clients feel about having an intravenous infusion?

● Do you control carefully the amount of intravenous fluid given during labour?

□ Acknowledgement

Figures 4.1 and 4.2 (on pages 63 and 64) are both taken from Macleod K G 1987 Analgesia and nutrition and the mother's choice in labour. Midwife, Health Visitor and Community Nurse 23 (9): 409–12. They are reproduced by kind permission of the Newbourne Group.

■ References

Beazley J M 1986 Natural labour and its active management. In Whitfield C R (ed) Dewhurst's textbook of obstetrics and gynaecology for postgraduates, 4th ed: Chapter 24. Blackwell Scientific, Oxford

Broach J, Newtown N 1988 Food and beverages in labor part II: the effects of cessation of oral intake during labor. Birth 15 (2): 88–92

Chez R A, Curcio F C 1987 Ketonuria in normal pregnancy. Obstetrics and Gynecology 69 (2): 272–74

DHSS 1989 Confidential enquiries into maternal deaths for England and Wales. HMSO, London

Douglas M J 1988 Commentary: the case against more liberal food and fluid policy in labor. Birth 15 (2): 93–4

Dumoulin J G Foulkes J E 1984 Commentary: ketonuria in labour. British Journal of Obstetrics and Gynaecology 91: 97–8

Evans S E, Crawford J S, Stevens I D, Drubin G M, Daya H 1986 Fluid therapy for induced labour under epidural analgesia: biochemical consequences for mother and infant. British Journal of Obstetrics and Gynaecology   93: 329–33

Guyton A C 1986 Textbook of medical physiology, 7th ed. W B Saunders, Philadelphia

Hazle N R 1986 Hydration in labour: is routine intravenous hydration necessary? Journal of Nurse-Midwifery   31 (4): 171–76

Hill G L, Blackett R L, Pickford I, Burkinshaw L, Young G A, Warren J V, Schorah C J, Morgan D B 1977 Malnutrition in surgical patients. Lancet   i: 689–92

Holdsworth J H 1978 Relationship between stomach contents and analgesia in labour. British Journal of Anaesthesia   50: 1145–48

Katch F I, McArdle W D 1983 Nutrition, weight control and exercise, 2nd ed: Chapter 3. Lea and Febiger, Philadelphia

Kenepp N B, Kumar S, Shelley W C, Stanley C A, Gabbe S G, Gutsche B B 1982 Fetal and neonatal hazards of maternal hydration with 5% Dextrose before Caesarean section. Lancet   i: 1150–2

Lancet 6th June 1987 Nutrition in sport. Lancet   i: 1297–7

Lewis M, Crawford J S 1987 Can one risk fasting the obstetric patient for less than 4 hours? British Journal of Anaesthesia   59: 312–14

Lind T 1983 Fluid balance during labour: a review. Journal of the Royal Society of Medicine   76: 870–75

Ludka L 1987 Fasting during labor. Paper presented at the International Confederation of Midwives 21st Congress in the Hague, August 1987.

Macleod K G A 1987 Analgesia and nutrition and the mother's choice in labour. Midwife, Health Visitor and Community Nurse   29 (9): 409–12

Mendiola J, Grylack L J, Scanlon J W 1982 Effects of intrapartum maternal glucose infusion on the normal fetus and newborn. Anesthetics and Analgesia   61: 32–5

Metzger B E, Ravnikar V, Vileisis R A, Freinkel N 1982 Accelerated starvation and the skipped breakfast in late normal pregnancy. Lancet   i: 588–92

Milner I 1986 Choosing a natural or an active childbirth. Nursing   3 (2): 39–45

Nimmo W, Wilson J, Prescott L F 1975 Narcotic analgesics and delayed gastric emptying during labour. Lancet   i: 890–93

Paterson P, Sheath J, Taft P, Wood C 1967 Maternal and foetal ketone concentrations in plasma and urine. Lancet   i: 862–5

Pearce J M, Steel S A 1987 A manual of labour ward practice: 14–5. John Wiley, Chichester

Power K J 1987 The prevention of acid aspiration (Mendelson's syndrome). Midwifery   3: 143–48

Pritchard J A, MacDonald P C, Gant N F 1985 Williams obstetrics 17th ed: 337. Prentice Hall, New Jersey

Robinson S, Golden J, Bradley S 1983 A study of the role and responsibility of the midwife. Chelsea College Nursing Research Unit, London

Simkin P 1986 Stress, pain and catecholamines in labour, 2: stress associated with childbirth events: a pilot survey of new mothers. Birth 13: 234–40

Tarnow-Mordi W D, Shaw J C L, Lin D, Gardner D A, Flynn F V 1981 Iatrogenic hyponatraemia of the newborn due to maternal fluid overload: a prospective study. British Medical Journal   283: 639–42

Thomas E A 1987 Pre-operative fasting – a question of routine? Nursing Times   83 (49): 46–7

Walia I 1986 Intranatal care in a rural community in Haryana, North India. Midwifery   2: 125

■ Suggested further reading

Birth volume 15 June 1988 Blackwell's Scientific Publications, 52 Beacon Street, Boston, Massachusetts 02108, USA

Evans S E, Crawford J S, Stevens I D, Drubin G M, Daya H 1986 Fluid therapy for induced labour under epidural analgesia: biochemical consequences for mother and infant. British Journal of Obstetrics and Gynaecology   93: 329–33

Hazle N R Hydration in labor. Journal of Nurse-Midwifery   31 (4): 171–76

Lind T 1983 Fluid balance during labour. Journal of Royal Society of Medicine   76: 870-75

Schearer M (ed) 1988 Birth   15 (2): whole issue

Chapter 5

Pain relief in labour

Alison M. Heywood and Elaine Ho

The aim of this chapter is to provide a theoretical and clinical background to pharmacological and non-pharmacological methods of pain control in labour. New insight is given into the range of methods which now exist so as to enable midwives to improve the choice of analgesics which they offer to women.

Since accurate and continuing assessment of pain for each client is essential to the decision on appropriate analgesia, the chapter opens with a review of the physiology of pain, an outline of pain theories and ways of measuring pain. The subsequent sections on pharmacological methods of analgesia aim to enable midwives to treat labour pain as promptly and effectively as the client desires.

Use of analgesia varies greatly, both from one country to another and from one establishment to another, depending on the prevailing philosophy and the expectations of the clients. In Britain up to a fifth of mothers use no recorded analgesia in labour (Heywood 1989) whilst mothers who do receive conventional analgesics are frequently dissatisfied, either with the degree of relief obtained or with the quality of their birth experience under the influence of drugs.

Midwives today may find that mothers in their care have knowledge of, and trust in, alternative methods of preparation and analgesia. Midwives may feel unable to support and advise the woman fully if they themselves are not familiar with a particular pain relieving technique and the mother may lose confidence in her attendants and feel that her preparation has been wasted.

The chapter discusses these non-pharmacological methods of analgesia in labour, the available literature about their efficacy and safety, and the amount of preparation necessary to use them successfully.

■ It is assumed that you are already aware of the following:

- The physiology of normal and abnormal labour;
- Fetal physiology, especially lung, cardiac and liver function;

- Modes of drug interaction and the nature of side effects experienced by mother and baby after the use of pharmacological modes of analgesia;

- Indications and contraindications for epidurals; the technique of 'topping-up';

- The UKCC rules (UKCC 1986a) relating to the giving of analgesia in labour by midwives.

■ The physiology of pain in labour

In order that midwives may help their clients to choose the most appropriate form of pain relief in labour, a clear and in-depth knowledge of the neuro-anatomy and physiology of pain is essential.

□ Innervation of the birth canal

The uterus, cervix and upper part of the vagina are innervated by the autonomic nervous system whilst the lower part of the vagina, the vulva, perineum and the pelvic floor muscles are supplied by the somatic nervous system. The pain of uterine contractions is transmitted by sympathetic nerve pathways to thoracic segments T10, T11 and T12. Sensations from the lower uterine segment and cervix (the pain of cervical dilatation) travel along the same pathways as the body of the uterus but may also be conveyed by the pelvic parasympathetic nerves (*nervi erigentes*) to enter the spinal cord at the second, third and fourth sacral segments. In the lower vagina, vulva, perineum and pelvic floor region, both sensory and motor impulses are conveyed by the pudendal nerves (with a contribution from the posterior cutaneous nerve of the thigh and the inferior pudendal nerve) and connect with the second, third and fourth sacral segments.

□ Types of nerve fibre

Nerve fibres can be classified into A delta, B and C fibres. The A delta fibres are myelinated somatic, the B fibres are myelinated autonomic and the C fibres are nonmyelinated autonomic and somatic fibres (Latham 1987). The two types of nerve fibres involved in pain transmission are the A delta and C fibres. The A delta fibres are grouped by size, the large fibres conducting at the fastest rate hence it is more difficult to suppress impulses passing down them (Shnider and Moya 1974). The A delta fibres are thought to give rise to sharp, well-defined localised pain while the thin, slow conducting C fibres produce diffuse, intense and unbearable pain.

☐ **Definition of pain**

Chapman (1977) conceptualises pain as a product of the individual's response to noxious sensory input as affected by the interactive influences of social/cultural, conceptual/judgmental, and emotional/motivational factors.

☐ **The physiology of pain**

The precise neurophysiological and biochemical mechanisms which cause pain during labour and delivery are inconclusive (Latham 1987). Pain during the first stage of labour is thought to be due to cervical dilatation and contraction of the myometrium (the latter causing ischaemic pain). The impulses travel along the sympathetic pathways to enter the spinal cord at the level of T10, T11 and T12. Like all visceral pain it is not well localised and has been described by mothers as 'cramp-like' or a 'deep ache' (Latham 1987). Pressure from one or more roots of the lumbosacral plexus and reflex skeletal muscle spasm may also result in pain. Once complete dilatation of the cervix is achieved pain is due to pressure and distension of the perineum and is conveyed by the pudendal nerves. As these are somatic nerves, sensation is well localised, sharp and intense. Impulses from uterine contractions will still cause pain in the lower abdomen and back.

☐ **Physiological effects of labour pain**

A summary of the possible effects of severe pain (caused by increased adrenaline secretion) is given in Table 5.1. Pain itself produces an increase in catecholamines and a decrease in uterine blood flow, therefore in fetal oxygenation. Catecholamines also decrease intrauterine pressure and hence the frequency and strength of contractions can be changed. Pain may also cause a labouring woman to hyperventilate; this can cause maternal alkalosis which has been found to induce fetal hypoxia (Levinson *et al* 1974). Narcotic analgesia and epidural analgesia can be effective in minimising pain along with hyperventilation and concomitant changes in blood gases (Crawford *et al* 1973; Riffel *et al* 1973; Belsey *et al* 1981).

■ Theories of pain

☐ **Specificity theory**

The specificity theory was one of the first efforts to develop a coherent physiological theory of pain (Von Frey 1894). It proposes that a specific

Table 5.1 Possible effects of severe pain

Severe pain dramatically increases adrenaline secretions causing:
- Increased cardiac output (from 15–60%)
- Increased heart rate
- Increased blood pressure
- Cardiac arrhythmias
- Severe hyperventilation leading to decrease in cerebral and uterine blood flow and fetal distress
- Alterations in function of uterus, gastrointestinal tract, kidney and urinary bladder
- Reflex spasm of skeletal muscles
- Nausea and vomiting

Severe pain also increases the body's level of catecholamines with a variety of physiological effects, and can decrease uterine blood flow leading to a reduction in fetal oxygenation

---

The information on which this table is based is derived from Read M D, Hunt L P, Anderton J P, Lieberman B A 1983 Psychological aspects of pregnancy. Longman, London

---

pain system carries messages from pain receptors in the skin to a pain centre in the brain. The theory goes on to propose that there are four major types of skin receptor, each sensitive to a specific stimulus (touch, cold, warmth and pain). Each type of receptor has its own projection system to the brain where it is interpreted in the centre responsible for the appropriate sensation (Latham 1987). Pain impulses are carried from free nerve endings scattered widely throughout the skin, subcutaneous tissues and viscera. The neural paths are made up of small, nonmyelinated C fibres which travel either through nerve trunks to the posterior roots of the spinal cord or through sympathetic nerve trunks to sympathetic ganglia and on to posterior roots of the spinal cord. One technique which has evolved from this theory is *nerve block*: for example pudendal nerve block is used to abolish the sensation of pain in the perineal, vulval and vaginal region during an instrumental delivery.

☐ **Two pathway theory**

This refinement of the original specificity theory became necessary when two different types and sizes of nerve fibres (A delta fibres and C fibres) were discovered to be involved in pain transmission (Head *et al* 1905). The A delta fibres are responsible for a sharp pricking type of pain while the C fibres carry a burning, intense pain. With this elaboration of the neuroanatomy and physiology, techniques for pain alleviation became more precise.

☐ Pattern or summation theory

'Patterning' or 'summation' describes the excitatory effects of converging inputs (Weddell 1955). When receptors normally activated by non-noxious heat or touch stimuli are subjected to excessive stimulations (that is summation of impulses) pain occurs because the total output of the cells exceeds a critical level. Hence, according to this theory, there are no specific pain pathways or nerve endings. Both noxious and non-noxious stimulation can lead to pain. For instance warmth can lead to heat which, as it increases in intensity, comes to be perceived as pain. This is true of cold, pressure, and other forms of non-painful stimulation.

☐ Central summation theory

This theory (Livingston 1943) attempts to explain phenomena such as phantom limb pain. It describes a central patterning of impulse flow, which creates for the patient a 'painful memory'. There is no peripheral stimulus as this has been withdrawn (for example by amputation). Instead a fixed pattern is locked into the central structures because it cannot be modified – as there is no normal sensory input from the original source.

☐ Gate control theory

This theory was conceived as an extension of the pattern theory (Melzack 1984a). Pain perception is the result of central and peripheral inputs, both of which act upon a 'gate' which controls the transmission of impulses to the pain centres of the thalamus and cerebral cortex. The gate is located in a portion of the dorsal column of the spinal cord. Peripheral input to the gate is conveyed by large A delta fibres and small C fibres. It is the combined influence of both inputs which influences the gate. To open this gate to pain perception a predominance of C fibre input must prevail. To close the gate to pain, A delta fibre input must predominate. The A delta fibres carry touch, pressure, and thermal stimuli, while C fibres carry cutaneous 'pain' and cold. Sustained impulses from type A fibres, such as impulses generated by TENS (see page 93), will inhibit transmission of pain to central cells.

☐ Endogenous opiate theory

This theory relates to the discovery of two types of neurotransmitters – the enkephalins and β-endorphins (Werle 1972). According to this discovery, the body manufactures opiate-like substances in order to provide pain relief at specific receptor-sites in the central nervous system. Enkephalins are found in the caudate nucleus, the anterior hypothalamus, and the substantia gelatinosa. They have a rapid-acting effect lasting about two minutes. The β-endorphin is found in the pituitary gland and has a four hour effect. It takes a larger pain stimulus – like labour pain – to activate the β-endorphin response.

☐ **Behaviourist theory**

This theory is based upon the idea that 'pain behaviours', such as grimacing, moaning or crying are all used to communicate pain (Fordyce 1973). These types of behaviours usually cause family members to sympathise and pay increased attention to the person displaying them. Thus, the behaviours themselves can become rewarding and inherently satisfying which can serve as a reinforcer for such behaviours. The treatment approach is to ignore pain behaviours in order to extinguish them gradually. It would, however, be quite inappropriate for a midwife to ignore a woman who is suffering from pain in labour.

■ Pain measurement

Ronald Melzack, one of the world's foremost authorities on pain, wrote that labour pain was one of the most controversial topics in the entire field of study (Melzack 1984a: 341). It clearly differs from many other forms of human pain, by its inevitable occurrence at the end of the gradual physiological process of pregnancy, by its intermittent pattern, rapidly rising to severe intensity and frequency, and by the expectation that it will vanish as soon as the infant is born. Contrast this with the timespan and intensity of pain from pathological conditions such as toothache, arthritis, cancer or postoperative pain.

Most primigravidae find labour pain the most excruciating experience they have ever endured, yet there are some who cope with no analgesia, and a few mothers who report no pain, or have such rapid labours that analgesia is almost irrelevant. The perfect analgesic for labour has yet to be discovered, so midwives need to gain an understanding of the techniques which may be used in trials of new analgesic methods, or evaluation of current ones.

Pain has been a subject of research for anaesthetists, physiologists, psychologists, midwives, nurses and physiotherapists. This research can be divided into two fields – clinical pain and its relief, and experimentally induced pain in healthy volunteers.

□ Experimental pain assessment

Various techniques may be used to test an individual's pain threshold, to judge the effectiveness of new medications and their antagonists at different dosages, and to see whether these parameters vary according to subjects' gender or age. The intensity of the painful stimulus may be measured subjectively or objectively. Subjective assessment, by the sufferer, includes verbal rating scales, pain questionnaires and visual analogue scales, discussed in more detail below. Objective measurement, by an observer, includes quantifiable physiological changes such as heart rate and blood pressure, dilation of pupils, sweating, facial expression and ability to concentrate on a task.

□ Clinical pain assessment

Clinical pain research has been extensive in the fields of postoperative pain, rheumatology, headache, back pain and cancer pain. The objective measures enumerated above are of interest in the detection of drug side-effects but it is generally held that subjective measurement of pain is the essential principal:

> Pain is whatever the patient says it is and exists wherever he says it does (Sternbach 1974).

Carers can certainly modify pain (and the effectiveness of analgesics) by the degree of sympathy, distraction, physical comfort and faith in treatment that they may be able to convey. They should *never* dismiss pain experienced by the patient merely because his prescription does not allow further medication yet, or his complaints seem inconsistent with the carer's expectations of a person with his diagnosis.

The most valid and widely used ways of assessing the subjective intensity of clinical pain are:

● The McGill Pain Questionnaire;

● Verbal ratings of
  – level of pain experienced,
  – degree of relief at intervals after analgesia,
  – intensity of any side-effects,
  – satisfaction with analgesia,
  – whether the same method would be chosen again;

● Visual or linear analogue scales.

A typical clinical trial would involve selecting a sample (for example sequential patients undergoing a particular operation), randomising them into a group to receive a known effective analgesic, a group to receive a new drug, and (if practicable) a group to receive a placebo medication. The trial should include enough patients to permit statistically significant results to be derived (at least 30 in each group) and should be conducted in a 'double-blind' fashion, that is neither the patients nor the staff administering the analgesia should be aware of which treatment is being given to any individual. The patients would be visited postoperatively by one of the research team (not involved in their daily care) and asked to rate their pain immediately before a dose of analgesia, and at, say, hourly intervals after each one. Crossover trials, where the groups of patients switch treatments after an appropriate exposure period, are not feasible in the case of pain of limited duration but may be used in studies of chronic pain such as the pain of arthritis.

☐ **Subjective pain measurement and its use in labour**

The McGill Pain Questionnaire, developed in Montreal in the 1970s (Melzack 1984a: 334–41), lists about 100 descriptive words from which the sufferer chooses those applicable to the type of pain presently experienced. These include 'scalding, heavy, flashing, drilling, terrifying, miserable, transient, rhythmic' and so on. The words are arranged in graded groups to measure sensory, affective, evaluative and temporal aspects of the pain, and the chosen words are later scored to give the sufferer's Pain Rating Index. The client is then asked to rank the pain on a verbal scale, as a measure of Present Pain Intensity:

0 no pain
1 mild pain
2 discomforting
3 distressing
4 horrible
5 excruciating

The whole questionnaire is usually read out to the client, taking about five minutes. It can also be self-administered.

Melzack (1984a: 342–3) used the questionnaire for 141 women in early labour and found that for both primiparae and multiparae the Pain Rating Index was, on average, higher than ratings given by patients suffering from cancer, phantom limb pain, post-herpetic neuralgia and other pain syndromes. Although multiparae generally gave lower ratings, 9 per cent of them and 25 per cent of primiparae reported their Present Pain Intensity as 'horrible' or 'excruciating' (note that this was still during early labour). The words most often chosen were 'sharp, cramping, aching, throbbing, stabbing, hot, shooting, heavy, tiring, exhausting, intense and tight'.

Melzack (1984a: 344–6) also studied the labour pain intensities of women taking different 'preparation for childbirth' courses and concluded that although preparation was of some value for primigravidae, there was scope for improving training methods, and women should always be informed about, and prepared to receive, forms of analgesia if necessary.

The McGill Pain Questionnaire is thorough, but undoubtedly too time consuming to administer to women in advanced labour. For convenience most investigators have used the Present Pain Intensity scale alone as a verbal score (often abridging it to 'no pain/mild/moderate/severe'), asked of the mother at half-hourly intervals. Instead, or in addition, a visual analogue scale (see Fig. 5.1) may be used. In this case the mother is shown a

Figure 5.1   10 cm visual analogue scale of pain intensity

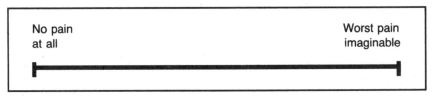

page with a 10 cm line, one end representing no pain, and the other representing the worst imaginable pain. She is asked to mark a point corresponding to the degree of pain felt during her last contraction. A new page is presented every half hour. This scale allows more choice in expressing degrees of pain than does a four or six point verbal score. The word 'analogue' in this context means an 'alternative representation' of pain severity (i.e. as a continuum rather than as steps).

Several problems with the above methods may occur in practice. Firstly individual contractions may vary in intensity so that the mother feels that her 'last contraction' was not typical. Secondly, unlike postoperative trials where the pain is initially severe and is expected to lessen, primigravid women cannot know how severe their pain may become. Some run out of space on the visual analogue line and place their marks at ever smaller intervals towards the right hand side. Labour pain is not only intermittent, but ever increasing, and if a woman insists that an analgesic has made no difference, this often passes unappreciated on the assumption that her pain would have become even worse without it.

Validation of these scales is described by Wallenstein (1984) who further presents complementary scales for relief of pain after analgesia (see Fig. 5.2). Other factors requiring regular monitoring are maternal pulse, blood pressure, frequency and strength of contractions, cervical dilatation etc. Effects on the baby can be monitored by fetal heart rate, colour of liquor, Apgar score and time taken until unaided respiration is established. Over the following days, neonatal measures such as weight gain (as a marker

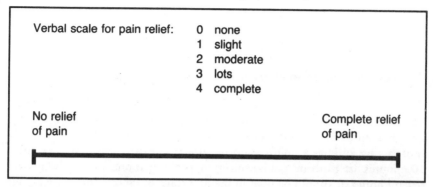

Figure 5.2 10 cm visual analogue scale of pain relief

of alertness/sucking behaviour), response to light and sound, and habituation to repeated stimuli (Brazelton 1973) are also noted. Biochemical tests on both mother and neonate are also common elements of studies.

A mother's postnatal evaluation of analgesia in labour is also invaluable. This can be obtained by asking her the following day to rate the method for efficacy and any side-effects, on scales such as excellent/good/fair/poor, and by asking if she would use the same method in a future labour (or recommend it to her friends).

Thus there are several means of regularly assessing a woman's pain in labour without the need for elaborate equipment. Some of the above scales may sound simplistic, but their application to conventional analgesics has resulted in surprising findings, such as Entonox providing better analgesia than pethidine (Holdcroft & Morgan 1974) and reduced maternal satisfaction following epidural analgesia (Morgan *et al* 1982b). There is clearly a need not only to evaluate new pain-relieving methods for their maternal and neonatal effects, but to re-examine current techniques to determine whether different administration methods (for example, client-controlled or continuous infusion techniques) would be beneficial.

■ Pharmacological methods of pain relief

□ Morphine

This was probably the first narcotic used for labour pain if opium is discounted. It has been used since the early 19th century and produces analgesia and some sedation. It also produces more neonatal respiratory depression than other narcotics such as pethidine. According to Goodman and Gilman (1965) the less pernicious effect of pethidine is due to its shorter duration of action. Also, morphine passes the blood-brain barrier of the neonate more readily than does pethidine (Goodman & Gilman 1965). For these reasons, morphine is seldom used today.

☐ Pethidine and its additives

Pethidine (Meperidine, Pamergan P100) was first synthesised over 40 years ago (Moir 1986). Pethidine is a narcotic agent, that is a powerful cortical analgesic and atropine-like antispasmodic (Bonta *et al* 1979) It is relatively short acting and has a mildly soporific effect. The drug begins to take effect 10 minutes after intramuscular injection, peaking at one and declining over several hours. It should be used in the first stage of labour and, once labour is established, as soon as the woman starts to feel pain which she wishes to be alleviated (Bunsden 1982). The dosage used is between 50 and 150 mg which may be repeated every four hours approximately. Pethidine may have side-effects such as:

- Nausea and vomiting due to the stimulation of the chemoreceptors trigger zone in the brainstem;

- Sweating and heat loss due to stimulation of the occulomotor nucleus;

- Contraction of smooth muscle in the bladder sphincters which can lead to retention of urine;

- Peripheral vasodilation mediated by histamine release and a fall in the activity of the sympathetic nervous system leading to a fall in cardiac output and blood pressure;

- Postural hypotension;

- Drowsiness and sleep;

- Slowing of the respiratory rate as the brain stem respiratory centre sensitivity to $PaCO_2$ is depressed.

Studies (Crawford *et al* 1973; Bundsen *et al* 1982) have shown that Apgar scores of 8 or less were more often observed after pethidine injections than when no pethidine was given.

See the section on naloxone (below) for details of reversing the effects of this drug.

☐ Pentazocine (Fortral)

Pentazocine is a synthetic analgesic which is not an opium derivative. Pentazocine 40 mg produces a comparable degree of analgesia to 100 mg pethidine and many women in labour will obtain satisfactory pain relief with 60 mg of pentazocine (Moir 1986). The drug crosses the placental barrier and in cases where this induces respiratory depression naloxone can be used as an antidote. The incidence of nausea and vomiting is lower than with pethidine (Moir 1986).

☐ **Phenothiazine derivatives**

The two phenothiazine derivatives in common use in labour are promethazine and promazine (Moir 1986). These are given intramuscularly in doses of 25 or 50 mg. They may be given with pethidine in which case it is usual practice to reduce the dose of the analgesic drug as phenothiazines tend to potentiate the effect of narcotic analgesics (Moir 1986). The phenothiazines do not depress respiration in the doses used in labour and uterine contractions are not inhibited (Mowat & Garrey 1970). Promazine may cause maternal and fetal tachycardia. Both promazine and promethazine have antiemetic and antihistamine actions. Both these drugs are contraindicated in women receiving antidepressants such as monoamine oxidase inhibitors and in women suffering from liver damage, symptomatic cardiovascular disorders and severe hypertension.

The use of a combination of promethazine and pethidine has enabled the dose of pethidine to be reduced by about 50 per cent and has resulted in more effective analgesia, sedation, shortening of labour and a decrease in neonatal depression (Riffel *et al* 1973). Riffel and colleagues also proposed that the increase in uterine activity may be due to the analgesic action of the drugs. To the extent that pain is associated with stress, its elimination in labour would decrease the release of adrenaline which is an inhibitor of uterine activity.

☐ **Meptazinol (Meptid)**

Meptazinol is an analgesic drug with partial opiate antagonist properties. It has little influence on cardiovascular and respiratory function in humans and no adverse effects in the newborn baby when given to the mother as an analgesic during labour (Sheikh & Tunstall 1986). The usual dose is 100 to 150 mg intramuscularly for pain relief in first stage of labour. It is better metabolised by the newborn baby and therefore claimed to be less likely to induce respiratory depression (Morgan 1982a). It is also likely to have an extremely low dependency producing potential.

Double blind studies (Nicholas & Robson 1982; Sheikh & Tunstall 1986; Osler 1987) comparing meptazinol and pethidine have found them to be of equal clinical value as analgesic injections during the first stage of labour.

☐ Naloxone (Narcan)

Narcotic antagonists are drugs that reverse the respiratory depression and analgesia in clients to whom narcotics have been given. Naloxone is the newest antagonist and was introduced into clinical medicine in 1971. (Bonta *et al* 1979). The usual dose for the newborn is 0.01mg/kg body-weight. The half life of naloxone is one hour with a duration of action of approximately 10–30 minutes.

Although women in labour benefit from the administration of narcotic analgesia, these drugs may affect the fetus and produce respiratory depression or subtle changes in alertness and general behaviour not reflected by Apgar scores (Bonta *et al* 1979; Belsey *et al* 1981). Studies (Hodgkinson *et al* 1978; Hodgkinson & Husain 1982) have shown that the elimination half life of pethidine is about 23 hours in the newborn and the pharmacological effect of maternally administered pethidine on the newborn is limited to the first three days following birth. Naloxone has been found to be valuable in reversing the respiratory depression in the neonate caused by pethidine given to the mother during labour (Bonta *et al* 1979; Welles *et al* 1984; Hibbard *et al* 1986). Bonta and colleagues (1979) suggest that the administration of naloxone should also facilitate recovery of neonatal alertness and normal suckling pattern.

☐ Epidural analgesia

The two forms of epidural analgesia used in obstetrics are lumbar epidural analgesia and caudal analgesia. The aim of the technique is to produce a selective block of the nerves from the uterus (T10, T11, T12 and L1) during the first stage of labour by giving an appropriate dose of bupivacaine (Marcain) with the woman in the horizontal position. When perineal pain is experienced the 'top-up' should be administered with the woman in the sitting position hence extending the block to the sacral roots (S2, S3 and S4). An effective top-up should take full effect in 10–15 minutes after injection and last between one and a half and two hours.

The local anaesthetic agent acts on the afferent sensory nerves within the epidural space. Bupivacaine is the most suitable anaesthetic agent and is available in 0.25 per cent, 0.5 per cent and 0.75 per cent strengths. The first two strengths are used in labour and the 0.75 per cent can be used for caesarean section. The administration of epidural pethidine and morphine has been studied but neither drug is considered advantageous in obstetric epidural analgesia (Husemeyer & Davenport 1981; Nybell-Lindahl & Carlsoan 1981). Bupivacaine becomes bound to maternal plasma protein, hence only about a fifth of the drug in the circulation crosses the placental barrier to the fetus. Studies have been carried out with respect to intramuscular pethidine and epidural bupivacaine on the influence of maternal

analgesia on neonatal behaviour (Belsey *et al* 1981; Rosenblatt *et al*
In this research neonates and adults showed different sensitivities to
drugs and displayed different effects. In both the pethidine and the
bupivacaine studies, however, it was found that the relationship between
maternal medication and infant behaviour was not a simple one. There was
no straightforward correlation between the amount of either drug given and
the observation of gross alterations in newborn function. Rather, the studies
suggest that the relationship is determined by the rate of change in the
concentration of a compound over time and also the rate the newborn's
ability to metabolise and excrete the drug.

Oakley (1980) links epidural analgesia to the postnatal 'blues' in her
study of transition to motherhood. A pharmacological link between drugs
used in epidural analgesia and emotional lability in the postnatal period has
not been established however (Read *et al* 1983). It has been suggested
(Murray & Dolby 1981; Rosenblatt *et al* 1981) that the effects of
bupivacaine on the newborn (such as poor visual and auditory response,
reduced alertness, reduced muscle tone and reduced activity) contribute to
the 'blues' by making the baby unresponsive to the mother in the critical
bonding period following birth.

Studies have been carried out to investigate the effects of epidural
analgesia on the progress of labour and some (Read *et al* 1983; Ogbonna &
Daw 1986) have shown that the effect of the epidural on length of labour is
dependent upon the time that it is given. According to Read and colleagues,
'there can be no reasonable doubt that epidural analgesia delays the
progress of labour particularly if it is given early in the latent phase'. They
further asserted that the incidence of instrumental deliveries is related to the
stage of labour at which epidural block is established. Chestnut *et al* (1988)
noted that epidural infusion of 0.125 per cent bupivacaine inserted or
'topped-up' beyond a cervical dilatation of 8 cm prolonged the second stage
of labour and increased the frequency of instrumental delivery in primigravidae. Studd *et al* (1982) present a slightly different view, claiming that
although a higher incidence of instrumental deliveries is associated with
epidural analgesia, cervical dilatation in the first stage of labour is not
affected by its administration. It could be that the relationship between the
increased rate in instrumental deliveries and epidural analgesia is a spurious
one. Crawford (1982) argues that cardiovascular dynamics influence intrauterine activity and suggests, therefore, that prevention of hypotension
and hypovolaemia during epidural analgesia will ensure uterine activity is
unimpaired and the duration of the first stage unaffected.

The effect of epidural analgesia on the duration of the second stage of
labour has been investigated. Bates *et al* (1985) postulated that with the
absence of Ferguson's reflex the force of uterine contractions in the second
stage is not increased and therefore a spontaneous delivery is less likely. The
length of time permitted for descent of the presenting part to the pelvic floor
is a controversial issue. Dorman and Wright (1983) argued that, provided

the fetal presenting part is low before expulsive efforts are made by the woman, there is a good chance of achieving spontaneous vaginal delivery even with epidural analgesia. Maresh *et al* (1983) and Buxton et al (1988) studied the effect of delayed pushing (that is women are encouraged to push only when the fetal, presenting part is visible at the vulva) in the second stage in women with effective epidural blocks. These studies showed no adverse effects on fetal acid-base balance. A study by Goodfellow and Hull (1983) indicates that the instrumental delivery rate in primigravidae may be decreased with oxytocic augumentation of the second stage. This is based on their finding that naturally occurring oxytocin levels were reduced due to absence of Ferguson's reflex in the group of women studied who had epidural analgesia.

Management of the second stage of labour will depend on the policy of the obstetrician and the anaesthetist. It may be considered useful to allow some sensation to return by giving lower doses of bupivacaine (Dorman & Wright 1983), however some researchers feel that after a pain free labour, such practice is unecessarily distressing to the woman (Crawford 1982).

□ **Epidural opiates**

Interest has focused recently on the efficacy of epidural opiates in relieving pain in labour. Hughes *et al* (1981) studied the effect of analgesia provided by the epidural injection of 0.5 per cent bupivacaine compared with that produced by the epidural injection of morphine in three doses (2, 5 or 7.5 mg) given to women during labour and at delivery. The 2 and 5 mg doses of epidural morphine did not produce satisfactory pain relief during labour, whereas 7.5 mg gave satisfactory relief during labour but not at delivery. Epidural administration of morphine, however, produces an unacceptable level of pruritus, urinary retention, nausea and vomiting (Abboud *et al* 1984a; Hughes *et al* 1981). Naloxone has been found to reverse these side-effects without affecting the analgesic effect of epidural morphine (Abboud *et al* 1984b).

Niv *et al* (1986) studied the analgesic properties and motor effect of epidural 0.25 per cent bupivacaine (8ml) compared with those of epidural morphine (2mg in 10 ml saline) followed by 8 ml of 0.25 per cent bupivacaine. Satisfaction with analgesia in the morphine-bupivacaine group was higher; pain relief lasted for a mean of 131.1 minutes (with a standard deviation of 49.8) as opposed to the plain bupivacaine group (a mean of 57 minutes with a standard deviation of 15.28). More significant is the finding that, in the morphine-bupivacaine group, good analgesia was obtained without such motor side-effects as weakness of the leg muscles.

The combination of epidural local anaesthetics and fentanyl has been demonstrated (Youngstrom *et al* 1984) to be beneficial in anaesthesia for labour and delivery. Because fentanyl has no effects on sympathetic or motor neurones, it provides certain advantages over local anaesthetics, but has been shown to be inadequate as the sole agent (Carrie *et al* 1981). There is evidence (Knepp *et al* 1983) that diluted solutions of bupivacaine in a larger volume are more effective than concentrated solutions in a small volume. Moreover, as diluted concentrations of bupivacaine have fewer motor effects, such combinations may be useful in reducing unpleasant effects (such as weakening of the leg muscles) and in reducing instrumental deliveries (Van Zundert *et al* 1984). Low concentrations of bupivacaine used alone will not, however, provide effective analgesia. Indeed, although lower concentrations of bupivacaine are sufficient to block the nonmyelinated C fibres in the first stage of labour they are not adequate in blocking the myelinated A delta fibres in the second state (Chestnut *et al* 1988). The combination of bupivacaine with fentanyl has been shown to result in longer and more effective analgesia with more rapid onset and longer duration (Celleno & Capogna 1988; Chestnut *et al* 1988). Heavy legs and loss of bearing down sensations are also avoided.

☐ **Continuous epidural analgesia**

Continuous epidural analgesia is now used widely to relieve pain in labour. During continuous epidural blockade the intermittent injection of local anaesthetic in response to the return of pain ('top-up' on demand) has been described as the method of choice in the belief that the total dose of local anaesthetic is minimised (Chestnut *et al* 1987). In a prospective comparative study (Purdy *et al* 1987) 240 women received epidural bupivacaine either by regular timed injections or 'on demand' for pain relief during the first stage of labour. In this study the quality and continuity of analgesia, motor blockade, spread of sensory blockade, cardiovascular changes and fetal outcome were recorded. Overall, the analgesia provided by regular 'top-up' injections was superior to the 'on demand' technique. This improved analgesia was achieved without compromise to the mother or the neonate. The only criticism is the fact that the study did not mention how the effect of analgesia was measured (for example by visual analogue carried out by the client or by observation by medical/midwifery staff). To maintain pain relief throughout labour, one or more incremental doses of local anaesthetic agent are usually required and this may be provided as regular 'top-ups' on demand. Each top-up may be preceded by a period of increasing pain for the woman and involves heavy demand on midwifery staff. The use of dilute local anaesthetics via an infusion pump has been found to provide women in labour with effective analgesia while keeping to a minimum of fluctuations of cardiovascular parameters after the establishment of the initial block (Faure *et al* 1980; Abboud *et al* 1984a; Bogod *et al* 1987). The risk of subdural migration of the catheter tip during the course of labour would suggest that the lowest concentration and dose of local anaesthetic agent compatible with significant prolongation of blockade should be used with such infusions. An infusion of 0.125 per cent bupivacaine (10 ml per hour) has been shown to be effective in maintaining analgesia in the first stage of labour without any adverse effects upon the mother and baby (Bogod et al 1987).

There is no doubt that a successful epidural block will provide total pain relief. Linblad et al (1987) asserted that, not only is epidural analgesia the most effective means of pain relief during labour, but it is also the type of obstetric analgesia that interferes least with the physiological response to labour in terms of its effect on fetal blood flow. Research has shown, however, that there is little correlation between pain relief and a satisfactory experience of labour. In Morgan's (1982a) study the epidural analgesia group included more women who felt their birth experience to be unsatisfactory than did the 'nitrous oxide and oxygen' or 'pethidine' groups where analgesia had been less effective. More important determinants appear to be the length of labour and the type of delivery the woman experienced. Kitzinger's (1988) study of 455 women in Britain and 453 women in Australia revealed that regrets and feelings of failure sometimes emerged weeks or months afterwards.

It is difficult to interpret studies of maternal satisfaction related to childbirth under epidural analgesia. Results will vary according to the woman's expectation of pain before labour as well as factors, such as pre-eclampsia, which may complicate labour. It is also important to bear in mind that Kitzinger's study was confined to a sample of women who were mostly members of the National Childbirth Trust and thus the sample was not selected randomly. Her results may not, therefore, be representative of the general population.

Kitzinger's (1988) study also highlighted the problem of ineffective pain relief, sudden drops in blood pressure and complications such as dural tap or accidental spinal anaesthesia. These complications were recognised in Crawford's (1986) study and in recent years there have been reports of serious maternal morbidity and mortality associated with obstetric epidural analgesia (Brahams 1982; Tomkinson et al 1982). Crawford asserted that among the safety features to be emphasised are the proper instructions to midwives in 'topping-up' procedures, well defined protocols for the management of complications, the immediate availability of resuscitation equipment and the in-house presence of an anaesthetist to attend the client within five minutes of identification of a problem over a 24 hour period. Hence it is disturbing to find in a study by Frank et al (1988) that only 16 out of 22 maternity units have a continuous anaesthetic back-up service, that instructions to midwives for 'top-ups' and subsequent care of women follow no uniform pattern, and that midwifery in-service training in the initial management of serious epidural complications and in cardiopulmonary resuscitation is inconsistent. In some units, the avoidance of aortocaval compression was not emphasised in the management of serious complications such as severe maternal hypotension, total spinal blockade or cardiac arrest. The authors sum up by claiming that their results suggest, 'there is a need to review the requirements in the provision of obstetric epidural services' and that 'consideration should be given to the establishment of a generally accepted standard of practice'.

☐ Epidural blood patch

Epidural blood patch is currently the accepted and definitive therapy for inadvertent dural puncture, but there has been considerable debate on the prophylactic use of this technique (that is treating all dural taps before they become symptomatic). Loeser *et al* (1978) reported a 71 per cent failure rate in the first 24 hours when they injected 10 ml of blood via the epidural catheter. In a more recent study, Ackerman and Colclough (1987) used the same technique and reported a 100 per cent success rate. The use of prophylactic epidural blood patch was further investigated by Cheek *et al* (1988) who treated 10 women by injecting 15–20 ml of autologous blood via an epidural catheter after inadvertent dural puncture. The time interval from dural puncture to prophylactic epidural blood patch ranged from 90 to 600 minutes. Their findings supported those of Ackerman and Colclough which suggest that prophylactic epidural blood patch is reliable in preventing post-lumbar headaches. They determined that the critical factor in assuming successful prophylactic epidural blood patch is the use of a sufficient volume of autologous blood (the lower limit may be 15 ml). Injection of blood through the epidural catheter, as opposed to directly through the epidural needle, does not appear to be important for success in prophylactic epidural blood patch. Opponents of the technique argue that formation of abscess and fibrinous arachnoiditis are serious potential complications, but if strict asepsis is maintained the incidence of infection should be very low.

☐ General anaesthesia versus epidural analgesia for elective caesarean section

From the mother's point of view, the outstanding advantage of epidural analgesia for caesarean section is that she can see and hold her baby at the time of birth. In many obstetric units the partner is encouraged to be present during delivery by caesarean section provided that it is carried out under epidural analgesia. If drug-induced respiratory depression occurs in the baby it is usually of such a low order as to be beyond the bounds of serious consideration (Crawford 1986). The possibility of respiratory depression in babies delivered under general anaesthesia is significant, especially if the fetus is not in optimal condition – for example if he is metabolically acidotic or suffers from intrauterine growth retardation.

Bupivacaine 0.5 per cent plain is the most commonly used agent for caesarean section under epidural block in Britain (Reid & Thorburn 1988). In 1984 Dutton *et al* studied the use of 0.75 per cent bupivacaine but found that it offered no advantages over 0.5 per cent bupivacaine plain. There appears to be a wide variation in the dosage of local anaesthetic agent required to produce an epidural blockade suitable for caesarean section (Dutton *et al* 1984).

The influence of maternal position on the epidural blockade produced for caesarean section is uncertain. Reid and Thorburn (1988) studied 64 women in either sitting or lateral position for elective caesarean section with either 0.5 per cent plain bupivacaine or 2 per cent lignocaine with adrenaline 1 in 200 000 in random allocation. They found that onset was shorter and a greater number of women were ready for surgery within 35 minutes following injection of local anaesthetic in the lateral position. Conversely the sitting position appeared to delay the spread of the upper limit of sensory blockage and prolong the time to readiness for surgery. Reid and Thorburn claimed that those sitting also required larger doses of the local anaesthetic but this failed to be statistically significant ($P < 0.05$). Nevertheless this highlights the need to study the influence of maternal position on the success of the epidural blockade as extensive blocks requiring a greater dose of local anaesthetic agents will inevitably induce hypotension (Dutton *et al* 1984).

Pretreatment with H_2 receptor antagonists to reduce gastric acidity before anaesthetics is becoming popular. Feely *et al* (1982) have shown that cimetidine (Tagamet) and ranitidine (Zantac) have different effects on the pharmacokinetic profile of lignocaine. They concluded that cimetidine decreases the clearance of lignocaine by inhibiting hepatic enzyme activity and decreases liver blood flow. This study has been criticised by Mitchell *et al* (1987) who suggested that methods of measuring liver blood flow have a significant margin of error. In a carefully designed random study Flynn *et al* (1989) investigated the effect of the H_2 antagonist pretreatment on the disposition of bupivacaine during epidural anaesthesia for caesarean section. This study shows that a single dose of cimetidine or ranitidine does not affect significantly the disposition of bupivacaine in pregnant women; however as there are only 30 women (that is 10 in each group of cimetidine, ranitidine and no treatment) these results cannot be generalised. Moreover plasma bupivacaine concentration is dependent not only on dose but also on rate of absorption, apparent rate of distribution and clearance. Antecedent variables such as age, weight and height of the clients should also be taken into account.

☐ **General anaesthesia**

It is beyond the scope of this chapter to deal with general anaesthesia in any great depth but certain pertinent issues will be discussed; the reader is directed to the 'Suggestions for further reading' at the end of this chapter for a thorough overview of general anaesthesia. The conflicting requirements of adequate oxygenation and minimal drug-induced respiratory depression in the fetus at delivery, and the avoidance of intraoperative maternal awareness and pain, present a dilemma in devising a general anaesthetic technique for caesarean section. The current use of an inspired anaesthetic gas mixture of 50 per cent nitrous oxide in oxygen with the addition of low concentration of volatile agents has not eliminated the problems (Reynolds 1986). It has been suggested (Reynolds 1986) that a brief and mild degree of neonatal sedation following delivery, caused by the use of higher concentrations of volatile gases such as ether or halothane, represents a minor disadvantage for decreasing the incidence of intraoperative awareness. This approach, however, has been criticised by Moir (1970) for it carries the increased risk of inducing maternal hypotension and inhibiting uterine contractions after delivery resulting in postpartum haemorrhage.

The techniques of general anaesthesia for caesarean section are devised to optimise neonatal condition at delivery, to produce maternal cardiovascular stability and to prevent maternal pulmonary aspiration. There is no doubt that further research is needed to enhance the techniques available. Bogod *et al* (1987) studied 40 women undergoing elective and emergency caesarean section. The study was designed to compare the effects of increasing the inspired oxygen concentration upon fetal oxygenation at a comparable depth of anaesthetic. For this to be possible, higher than usual inspired concentration of volatile agents are required. As a result of the study, the researchers proposed a technique involving the use of higher inspired oxygen concentration which they claim is safe, having no effect on uterine contractility and blood loss. Moreover the depth of anaesthesia produced ensured that no women reported awareness or recollection of the operation.

A common cause of mortality and morbidity attributable to anaesthesia is difficult or failed intubation. In obstetric anaesthesia, 2.7 per cent of intubations are reported to be difficult and the estimates for failed intubation are 0.05–0.3 per cent (Lyons & MacDonald 1985). If the women in whom intubation proves difficult could be identified in advance, it could be arranged for an experienced anaesthetist skilled at dealing with such problems to be present. Wilson *et al* (1988) tried to assess 633 adult patients undergoing routine surgery in order to formulate a predictive index based on five risk factors (weight of patient, head and neck measurement, degree of jaw movement, degree of mandibular recession and number of buck teeth). This index was subsequently tested prospectively on 778 women and detected 75 per cent of women who were difficult to intubate. There was a 12 per cent false positive rate which is unacceptable as this would increase unnecessary calling of skilled assistance thus depleting scarce resources. This study nevertheless highlights the inadequacy of current attempts to predict difficult intubation and to ensure that there is a clear policy for intubating those who may prove difficult.

☐ **Paracervical and pudendal blocks**

Paracervical and pudendal blocks are used frequently in many parts of the world where obstetric anaesthetists are not available. The duration of pain relief varies with the type of local anaesthetic, and its concentration and the total dose. It also varies widely among different parturients. With 0.25 per cent bupivacaine, relief is found to last about 90–150 minutes (Gottschalk & Hamilton 1975). The addition of epinephrine 1:400 000 was found to increase duration by about 25 per cent. This not only causes local vasoconstriction, however, it may also cause systemic effects consisting of adrenergic stimulation resulting in an increase in heart rate, stroke volume, and greater decrease in diastolic pressure resulting in shock (Bonica *et al* 1971). The enzyme hyaluronidase has also been advocated as an adjuvant to local anaesthetics by Gottschalk and Hamilton (1975) who claim it accelerates the spread of anaesthetic solutions to which it is added.

☐ **Inhalation analgesia**

The inhalant analgesia approved for use by midwives in Britain (UKCC 1986a) is a mixture of 50 per cent nitrous oxide and 50 per cent oxygen given via the Entonox apparatus. Analgesia is effective in 15–30 seconds as pulmonary transfer is rapid, with no residual effect detectable one minute after cessation of inhalation. The woman should be taught to inhale the gas as soon as she feels her uterus harden and to continue until the peak of the contraction has passed. This form of analgesia is usually used at the end of the first stage of labour. It can also be used as an adjunct to systemic analgesics – for instance before pethidine starts to take effect. Its main advantages are that it has a rapid action with no cumulative or adverse effects such as respiratory depression in the mother or neonate, it does not interfere with uterine contractions, it is not contraindicated in women with cardiac or pulmonary disease and, in addition, it is self-administered and therefore under the woman's control.

In one study investigating pain relief during labour (Bundsen 1982), clients were randomly allocated to three different groups. One group received epidural analgesia, one group was given both intravenous pethidine and inhalation analgesia and one group was given pethidine intramuscularly and inhalation analgesia. Pain relief was considered satisfactory by 88 per cent in the epidural group, by 53 per cent in the intravenous pethidine/inhalation analgesia group and by 67 per cent in the intramuscular pethidine/inhalation analgesia group. Another study (Harrison *et al* 1987) showed that the use of 50 per cent nitrous oxide and 50 per cent oxygen via the Entonox machine provided optimum pain relief to women if used correctly, that is, commencing inhalation with the onset of contractions and in the second stage by anticipating the onset of contractions. Instruction by the midwife is needed to achieve this. The same study also revealed that the 20 women using 50 per cent nitrous oxide and 50 per cent oxygen had the shortest labour and consequently expressed satisfaction with this form of analgesia. The authors however did not discuss whether the short duration of labour was the reason why these women did not request other types of analgesia.

The average exposure of midwives to nitrous oxide in delivery suites which did not have an active ventilation system was found in one study (Munley *et al* 1986) to be above 100 parts per million (PPM). Differences in working practices and in the layout, size and ventilation of delivery suites contributed to the observed differences in the average exposure. In one hospital the average exposure was 360 PPM, reduced by a factor of about 2.5 when a trial scavenging system was used. These results emphasised the importance of proper ventilation. Theoretical calculations show that the National Institute for Occupational Safety and Health's standard of 30 PPM for nitrous oxide could be achieved only by room ventilation with 32 changes of air per hour, but Munley and colleagues (1986) argued that this is not reasonable practice. They did recommend, however, that in every delivery suite, regular checks of performance should be carried out to ensure that the ventilation system is achieving an average of less than 100 PPM in all areas.

Lowe's (1987) study on individual variation in the pain of childbirth suggests that pharmacological methods of pain relief are only part of the answer. Other variables influencing women's experience of pain include preparation for childbirth, parity, anxiety level, the woman's confidence in her ability to cope with labour, concern regarding the outcome of labour for herself and her baby, and fear of pain itself. Midwives must recognise the importance of 'empowering' women (see the chapter by Sheila Drayton in this volume, 'Midwifery care in the first stage of labour', especially pages 27–32) and enhancing their self confidence. They also have an important role in helping clients to chose the most appropriate pharmacological and non-pharmacological methods of pain relief to suit their individual requirements. In order to help readers fulfil this latter role, the remainder of this chapter explores lesser known and non-pharmacological methods of pain relief in labour.

■ Non-pharmacological methods of pain relief

Alternative methods of pain relief include transcutaneous electrical nerve stimulation (TENS), acupuncture, homoeopathy, herbalism, massage techniques, hypnosis and active birth preparation. The latter, and the related techniques of yoga, controlled breathing, relaxation training and water baths to aid labour, will not be dealt with in depth, as their benefits are evident to most midwives. Influential authors have included Flynn *et al* (1978), concerning ambulation, Mendez-Bauer (1980) on upright posture, and Milner (1988) on bathing during the first stage of labour. Position in the second stage of labour is covered in the chapter 'Spontaneous delivery' by Jennifer Sleep in this volume. Psychoprophylaxis is reviewed in current midwifery and obstetric textbooks, and Heyns' abdominal decompression apparatus, promoted in the late 1950s, has fallen into disuse in Britain after reports of complications and is not dealt with here.

Aspects of the environment that may reduce anxiety and pain and help a woman to feel in control of her labour should not be forgotten. Subdued lighting, music, home-like birthing rooms (with equipment available behind curtains or outside until needed), privacy, choice of companion, constant sympathetic attendance when required – all of these are attainable in any hospital and may do much to enhance a mother's perception of her labour and reduce reports of pain. The vital role of a supportive labour companion in reducing a woman's analgesic requirements (Rosen 1977) has recently been re-affirmed (O'Driscoll & Meagher 1986). The experience of many community and independent midwives is that analgesics are rarely required, even for primigravidae, when care has been given on a one-to-one basis during pregnancy (Weig 1984; Sakala 1988).

The alternative techniques described below are either omitted or mentioned fleetingly in recent textbooks. The following sections give a practical account of each method, consider their availability, and discuss research findings where applicable, so that midwives may understand the scope of each, and be able to advise mothers accordingly. To those familiar with some of these therapies, the descriptions may still seem superficial, but further information is available from the sources listed, and a list of pertinent organisations is also given at the end of the chapter.

With the exception of TENS, these non-pharmacological methods are based on holistic philosophy, which states that the mind, body and spirit should be treated as a whole. A therapist should take time to talk through many aspects of a client's lifestyle, because the treatment chosen will depend on general wellbeing, as well as on the presenting symptoms. Most of these techniques emphasise general health promotion and, rather than claiming to provide analgesia for acute pain in labour, they aim to prepare the body (and mind) by conditioning or 'tonifying' it. It seems fair to observe that such measures will appeal mainly to women with a predisposition towards 'alternatives' – those who are prepared actively to seek out such advice and spend the appropriate time in preparation.

Despite regular criticism by the medical establishment that such therapies are a waste of time, ineffective or even heathen, many women using alternative methods do very well in labour. It should be remembered that the placebo effect of 'inert' substances is an accepted fact in analgesic research, and is particularly influenced by psychological factors, including the attitudes of staff. Further evaluation would certainly be valuable for alternative therapies, but there are obvious problems in undertaking randomised controlled trials in the way that they are used for pharmaceutical analgesics. Acupuncture, for instance, could hardly be administered to a client in a double blind trial against an injection or tablet, without her knowing which treatment she was receiving.

☐ **Transcutaneous electrical nerve stimulation**

Abbreviated variously to TENS, TNS or even TES, this technique has been promoted increasingly for obstetric use over the past 15 years. Its use by physiotherapists and anaesthetists (especially in pain clinics) goes back much further, and there is a historical precedent in an ancient Roman treatment in which a painful limb was intentionally stung by an electric fish to produce numbness. Excessive claims made for electrotherapy of all types in the 19th century resulted in its disuse; its recent revival for analgesia has been attributed primarily to Melzack and Wall's (1965) gate control theory.

TENS has been used successfully for chronic conditions such as phantom limb pain, post-herpetic neuralgia, painful joint conditions, and more acute conditions such as sports injuries and postoperative analgesia (Baxter 1983; Woolf 1984). Trials on postoperative patients have shown that functioning TENS units produced a 77 per cent relief of pain compared with the 33 per cent placebo effect of sham TENS units (see below), and significantly decreased the patients' narcotic requirements (Woolf 1984).

Earliest reports of obstetric TENS in the medical press are found in the late 1970s (Augustinsson *et al* 1977; Robson 1979; Stewart 1979), and interest has spread with the publication of case studies (Gowers 1985; Keenan *et al* 1985; Pickles 1987), practical recommendations for teaching about TENS (Polden 1984, 1985) and articles in women's magazines.

Obstetric TENS stimulators are dual-channel and usually priced between £100 and £250 (1989 UK prices). The most significant development has been a patient control or booster switch, enabling the stimulation to be switched between a low background level and a higher intensity for use during contractions. Many hospitals now have such machines and a few companies and lay childbirth groups have initiated short term hire schemes.

The basis of TENS is square-wave pulses of electricity produced by a small portable stimulator. Manufacturers' instructions often describe low and high 'intensity' or 'stimulation', but there are actually three parameters of the current to be considered. These are the amplitude (height or intensity) of each pulse, the frequency (the number of pulses per second, called Hertz or Hz), and pulse width (the time span of each pulse). Most obstetric stimulators have a pre-set pulse width, at a value between 80 and 200 microseconds, as this has been found to be the most comfortable and effective range. The amplitude and frequency are altered by dials to suit the individual and to achieve a strong but comfortable tingling sensation. By adjusting the frequency the woman can choose anything from a throbbing or ticklish feeling to a smooth floating sensation. The amplitude usually needs increasing occasionally, as the contractions intensify and the body becomes accustomed to the stimulation.

The booster switch or slider raises the level of stimulation, by switching from 'pulse train' mode (which is also referred to as 'pulse burst' or 'acupuncture-like TENS') to a 'continuous' stream of pulses, or to a higher amplitude or frequency, depending on the design. Used during contractions this should reduce transmission of pain signals rapidly, in accordance with the gate control theory. The background pulse train mode stimulates release of endorphins, rising during the first half hour of use (Salar *et al* 1981). Both of these explanations have their critics. Some aspects of the gate control theory have been discredited, but no better explanation of short term TENS analgesia has emerged (Woolf 1984). Endorphins are produced naturally in response to fear, stress and excitement, so an increase is to be expected due to labour itself (Bonica 1984).

☐ **Practical and safety aspects of TENS**

Obstetric stimulators have two channels and four electrode pads are used. Reusable carbon rubber electrodes about 4 cm by 10 cm are the most economical, and may be applied to the skin by several means, provided good conductive contact is achieved. The recommended sites for labour are dorsal. One pair of pads are placed at the level of T10–L1, and the other at the level of S2–S4, about 5 cm on either side of the spine. These overlie the roots of the afferent nerves serving the uterus and cervix and the vagina and perineum respectively.

Research is continuing on the safety and merits of abdominal electrode placement (for example over the iliac fossae) when the pain is primarily suprapubic. The analgesic effect does not seem to be consistently improved, and electrical interference with cardiotocographs may be more likely (see below), but there is no risk of affecting the fetal heart rate at the usual current densities (Bundsen & Ericson 1982).

TENS is most useful if started early in labour, and ideally the woman will have had the chance to try it out beforehand. The dorsal sites are suitable, near term, to indicate the sensations obtainable during labour; alternatively the forearm can be used, although there are more nerve endings here and the effect is rather more 'prickly'. Many women, though, have used TENS successfully without any antenatal practice, even if they haven't started using it until labour is advanced. Its best effect is seen in women with back pain, especially multigravidae, who wish to remain ambulant.

TENS alone may not give sufficient analgesia for the later stages of labour, but its continued use may enable a woman to use less conventional analgesia and to feel more in control (see the 'Recommendations for clinical practice' on page 110).

In view of the observation that some modalities of acupuncture and TENS can shorten labour, there is a theoretical risk of stimulating contractions. It is advised, therefore, that TENS should not be tried on the back or abdomen before 37 weeks gestation. It has, however, been used safely throughout pregnancy on other sites to control sciatica and carpel tunnel syndrome. To date, no side-effects have been found in either mother or baby.

TENS is contraindicated for people with demand-type cardiac pacemakers; the only other medical cautions are in relation to use over the eyelids or upper chest (irrelevant for obstetrics). It cannot be used while a woman is in the bath. TENS machines always use batteries, not mains electricity, and well designed machines would cut out in the event of a short circuit or power surge.

A much quoted problem is electrical interference with cardiotocograph (CTG) equipment. This has been reported in about 50 per cent of cases with fetal scalp electrode monitoring (Bundsen *et al* 1981), but in only one isolated case with external (ultrasound) monitoring (DHSS 1987). Possible symptoms of such interference are superimposed blips on the trace, a spurious high frequency readout mimicking a persistent tachycardia, no fetal heart rate display, or intermittent 'scratchiness' of the trace, usually during contractions when the TENS booster switch is activated. This interference seems dependent upon the particular combination of CTG and TENS machines, so the problem may never be encountered in some hospitals.

The possibility of transmission problems such as a loose scalp electrode must first be eliminated. Proof of TENS interference is readily accomplished by switching the TENS unit off completely for a couple of contractions and observing the tracing, which will return to normal if TENS was the sole problem.

It is always possible to hear the true fetal heart rate from the monitor or by auscultation, and annotation of the tracing to this effect may be sufficient in low risk cases. Interference may be minimised or eliminated by altering the position of the TENS electrodes or the stimulator itself, or decreasing the level of stimulation (DHSS 1987). Otherwise, a clinical decision must be taken as to whether a clear CTG readout or the use of TENS is more important at that time. Progress has been made to filter out such signals from the CTG trace or to devise different electrodes (Bundsen & Ericson 1982). It is emphasised that there is no question of the fetal heart rate itself being affected by the TENS, only the electronic monitoring of it.

□ **Research concerning TENS in labour**

A number of trials have been reported, some of which are summarised in Table 5.2 and those of note are then discussed in more detail. In brief, safety

Table 5.2   Summary of selected studies on TENS analgesia in labour

Author & date	Number using TENS		Good Analgesia obtained		Remarks
	PO	P1+	PO	P1+	
Augustinsson et al 1977	90	57	48%	37%	Further 44% had moderate pain relief. Suprapubic pain often helped by sacral stimulation
Robson 1979	13	22	54%		6 multiparae & 1 nullipara used no other analgesia
Stewart 1979	34	33	79%	79%	All but 5 multiparae used some additional analgesia
Bundsen et al 1981		283	38% (for low back pain)	38%	Versus <20% for controls with other analgesia. ? Shorter labours. Apgar scores better
Tawfik et al 1982	35	–	53%	–	No additional analgesia used – 55 controls had pethidine only. Shorter 1st stage and better Apgar scores in TENS group
Merry 1983		9	78%		Control group of 8 had sham TENS, with similar results to real TENS (see text)
Grim & Morey 1985	11	4	87%		Pethidine used by 8 women; reduced dosage. TENS subsequently used on 150 women: good or moderate relief for 80%
Stewart 1986	–	12	–	100%	2 of 12 in control group had pethidine, Entonox used by 8 controls & 10 TENS users
Harrison et al 1986	49	23 (all P2)	77%	81%	As judged postnatally. Placebo group gave worse scores postnatally but similar scores in labour to real TENS users

Notes:
1. PO = nulliparae, P1+ = multiparae; the figures are pooled if so given by the original author
2. 'Good analgesia obtained' = percentage of subjects reporting TENS to be very or moderately helpful: some authors gave limited scales such as 'excellent/fair/no help', so please see originals for details of protocols

has been confirmed, pain relief has been variable, labours have sometimes been shorter and most mothers have been very satisfied retrospectively with their labours. The effect of TENS alone is difficult to determine, however, as in most studies the mothers were recruited from amongst those who had already expressed an interest, they were able to use conventional analgesia concurrently if needed, control groups were difficult to define and good Apgar scores were often taken as sufficient evidence of safety. 'Conventional analgesia' varies considerably with the country of study. Bundsen *et al* (1981) give a cogent explanation of why neither prior randomisation of women nor restriction of supplementary analgesia were feasible in their large study. In three of the studies (Robson 1979; Grim & Morey 1985; Stewart 1986) some women acted as their own controls when the TENS units were turned off for several contractions during the first stage of labour. The authors note that such mothers were more distressed during this period and anxious to resume TENS – which appears to lend support to the gate control and/or distraction component of the effect of TENS.

Studies using TENS in a double-blind fashion have only been possible where the labour ward staff have no prior knowledge of the technique so cannot tell whether women are receiving real TENS or placebo. Either some of the machines need to be nonfunctioning (so that the indicator light still flashes but no current passes through the electrodes) or, to test the gate control component, the electrodes could be placed elsewhere than over the painful sites and relevant nerve roots. Merry (1983) carried out such a study, using real TENS on nine mothers and sham TENS on eight. Over half the women in each group later required pethidine or epidural block, although slightly more of those using real TENS reported that it was 'some help'. The report does not mention any booster facility. Other factors which may have contributed to sub-optimal results were the small electrodes used, their wide placement away from the spine, and the limited verbal pain relief scale (excellent, some help or useless).

In a much larger study, Harrison *et al* (1986) randomly allocated 150 consenting women who had not already decided on a specific form of analgesia to one of six TENS stimulators, three being 'placebo' machines. Measurements of initial pain threshold, hourly scores for pain and degree of pain relief, obstetric outcome, Apgar scores and cord blood pH all showed no significant differences between those using real or placebo TENS. In both parity groups, however, significantly more women using real TENS completed their labours with the sole addition of Entonox, rather than pethidine or epidural analgesia. In addition postnatal assessment of analgesia was more favourable amongst mothers (and their midwives) who had used real TENS machines. The authors took care that neither the midwives nor the mothers could distinguish the placebo TENS units; however, since TENS stimulation should ideally be at an intensity just below the individual's pain threshold, it seems doubtful whether mothers with real TENS units were using them optimally, otherwise their comments about the sensation might have alerted staff. Although further analgesia was required for the majority, the authors conclude that consumer satisfaction was such that TENS would be worth pursuing with machines specifically designed for labour. Such a development was in fact already under way with the advent of the booster switch described earlier.

Bundsen *et al* (1981) conducted the largest study to date, by offering TENS to all women with potential vaginal deliveries in one year (a take up rate of 283 out of 2683 total deliveries). Each was matched with the woman delivering nearest in time to her, of comparable parity, age and cervical dilatation on admission. Other methods of analgesia were used as required and all the study mothers completed a questionnaire about two hours after delivery. Over twice as many mothers in the TENS group (as opposed to the control group) reported good relief of low back pain. Epidural analgesia was rarely used. The great majority of mothers in both groups used Entonox and/or pethidine, but TENS mothers used Entonox less often than those in the control group. Considering all forms of analgesia together, good relief of suprapubic pain was only achieved by 11.5 per cent of mothers. Primigravidae receiving TENS were more likely to wish to have the same analgesia in a future labour, and their babies had better Apgar scores and were less likely to need transfer for neonatal observation (although the general use of such observation seems high at over 25 per cent).

The study which examined possible side-effects on the fetus/neonate most thoroughly was also by Bundsen *et al* (1982). This only included 14 women using TENS, all with induced labours, and almost all of whom used additional analgesia. They were compared with a control group of 10 women using conventional analgesics. Extensive fetal assessment and biochemical and neurobehavioural tests on the neonates were carried out. No adverse effects of TENS were found. All values were comparable to those in other studies of induced and spontaneous births.

One study specifically aimed to quantify the effect of TENS compared with the standard labour analgesic, pethidine. Tawfik *et al* (1982) compared 35 Egyptian primigravidae using TENS alone with 55 having pethidine 50 mg intramuscularly, repeated 4–5 hourly if required. Personal support with relaxation and controlled breathing were emphasised generally, and all women received a routine intramuscular dose of diazepam 10 mg at the start of labour. TENS was considered statistically comparable to a total mean dose of 93.6 mg pethidine, and free of maternal side-effects, whilst 15 of the pethidine group experienced drowsiness, nausea or vomiting.

☐ **Indications for use of TENS**

The maternity units using TENS most successfully tend to be those where its introduction has involved collaboration between midwives, physiotherapists and medical staff, and where enough machines are available for mothers who have expressed an interest antenatally to be assured of the chance to use TENS in labour. TENS has also proved beneficial in alleviating postoperative and perineal pain, after pains, and the often distressing contractions felt after vaginal prostin insertion for induction of labour. It remains difficult to predict which mothers will do well with TENS, but there is nothing to lose by offering TENS to any suitable client, especially ambulant multiparae with back pain in labour (as mentioned above). If TENS is limited to interested primigravid parentcraft attenders it will take many months before each midwife feels competent in its use.

In Britain some maternity units restricted the use of TENS after the UKCC (1986b) reaffirmed that midwives should not use TENS equipment on their own responsibility but only under medical supervision. Midwives must of course be trained and feel competent in any treatment they carry out, and TENS training can be accomplished in one or two practical sessions, possibly with the involvement of an obstetric physiotherapist or anaesthetist. Many units have taken the approach of adding TENS to a 'standing order' list of items approved by the medical staff for use by midwives. Others sanction the application and adjustment of TENS therapy by a physiotherapist or the woman's partner.

□ **Acupuncture**

Acupuncture (this Western name being derived from the Latin for 'needle-pricking') is an ancient system of medicine, both preventive and curative, used extensively in the Far East. Only in Finland has it been incorporated into standard medical training. Western schools of acupuncture emphasise differing aspects, some providing short courses for health professionals to learn circumscribed techniques for limited purposes, others maintaining that an understanding of the totality of Traditional Chinese Medicine is essential. Some associations accept only doctors (often anaesthetists special-ising in pain control), others are open to non-medically qualified acu-puncturists, and their membership includes a number of midwives and physiotherapists. These bodies all organise training and certification of practitioners, but at present it is not illegal for an individual to describe him or herself as an acupuncturist without any formal training.

The traditional philosophy states that good health relies on the correct balance of Yin and Yang (positive and negative forces) throughout the body. To maintain the balance, life energy ('Qi' or 'Chi') should flow freely through the 14 'meridians' running through the torso to various peripheral points on the body. The meridian channels reflect particular internal organs (for example the heart, the spleen, the large intestine), although their existence has so far eluded orthodox anatomists.

Diagnosis in the traditional system involves detecting imbalances in the flow of energy through the meridians by sensing these at six pulse points on each wrist, together with a thorough history and physical examination. Therapy consists of several treatments at intervals of days or weeks, the practitioner inserting maybe four to ten needles into specific points along the meridians to facilitate the energy flow.

The very fine sterile needles are pushed in until a heavy numb feeling ('teh chi') is obtained in the area. To achieve this they may be twirled or twitched, either manually or by an electrical stimulation machine, at a pulsation rate of 2–4 per second, thought to encourage endorphin production. Typically, the needles are left in position for half an hour. A variation in treatment is *moxibustion* – the smouldering of a small quantity of moxa herb (mugwort or *artemisia vulgaris*) over the acupuncture point. Related therapeutic modes treat the same acupuncture points by massage (acupressure or Shiatsu; see Box 1984) or, recently, by laser.

A further development has been the auriculotherapy system propounded in the past few decades by the French doctor, Paul Nogier (Lewith 1982). In this system the human body is held to be mirrored in the shape of the ear (similar to an inverted fetus) and acupuncture with shorter needles or semi-permanent studs may be used at appropriate points on the pinna. Similarly, in reflexology (see below) regions such as the foot or hand have therapeutic points described, stimulation of which affects distant areas.

In Chinese medicine acupuncture has been used for minor pregnancy disorders, to correct fetal malpresentation (Bendiner 1985) and recently to induce labour and to provide anaesthesia for caesarean section. In the West, acupuncture has been used primarily to alleviate pain in such conditions as migraine headaches, joint and neuralgic pain, and also to combat smoking, drug addiction and obesity. Its application to labour pain is relatively recent.

Reports of acupuncture anaesthesia in the Far East have sounded very impressive – for example Meiyu (1985) reporting that 98 per cent of caesarean sections in one hospital are carried out under acupuncture – but have been criticised by Skrabanek (1984) and others as misleading in that premedication, local anaesthetics and narcotics are commonly used as adjuncts. No extra medication has been used, though, in reported operations on cattle under acupuncture anaesthesia (BMA News Review 1984).

Acupuncture's pain relieving effect is thought to be due to the production of endorphins, but neither this nor the gate control theory explains its long term analgesic effects, nor its effectiveness for diseases such as asthma and ulcerative colitis. The possible mechanisms are discussed by Melzack (1984b), Skelton and Flowerdew (1985) and Lewith (1982). Melzack holds that transmission via nerves rather than meridians is fundamental to effective pain relief from acupuncture, quoting studies involving reversal of analgesia with naloxone, blocking by procaine injection, animal experiments with neurotransmitters, and failure of acupuncture analgesia in the torso when acupuncture was applied to the legs of paraplegics. To achieve analgesia an induction time of about 20 minutes is typical and Melzack concludes that intense stimulation, rather than the precise site, is the essential element in this type of analgesia.

Traditional charts show over 360 effective acupuncture points along the meridians and it has recently been found that many of these coincide with areas of low electrical skin resistance. Trigger points (which can be stimulated by finger pressure) and motor points (where the greatest density of motor nerves serving a muscle occurs) have also been found to have similar distributions to acupuncture points (Melzack 1984b). The significance of these observations has not been fully elucidated.

□ Research studies involving acupuncture

As with TENS, controlled trials of acupuncture are few, but clinical reports from several countries are summarised in Table 5.3. A pilot study was carried out in Sri Lanka by Perera (1979); women admitted at term for induction (artificial rupture of membranes and oxytocin intravenous infusion) were offered acupuncture analgesia. The take up rate is unspecified

Table 5.3 Summary of trials on acupuncture in labour

Author & date	Number using Acupuncture		Good analgesia obtained		Effect on duration of labour	Remarks
	PO	P1+	PO	P1+		
Abouleish & Depp 1975	12		58%		None	Electro-acupuncture: safe, but analgesia inconsistent & incomplete
Vallette *et al* 1976	31		71%		No comment made	Good for posterior fetal positions
Kubista & Kucera 1976	20		25%		None	Moderate analgesia in a further 30%
Hyodo & Gega 1977	16	16	60%	90%	Shorter 2nd & 3rd stage	
Perera 1979	38	22	89%	95%	Shorter for all parities	ARM & oxytocin IVI used for all women. Control group: longer labours
Umeh 1986	14	16	64%	62%	None	Sacral needles
Lyrenäs *et al* 1987a	56	–	20%	–	Similar to controls	NB acupuncture given antenatally only
Skelton & Flowerdew 1988	34	49	26%	80%	1st stage shorter	This benefit only seen in primigravidae with normal labours and deliveries (n=8)

Notes:
1. PO = nulliparae, P1+ = multiparae; the figures are pooled if so given by the original author
2. 'Good analgesia obtained' = percentage of subjects reporting 'excellent/very good/good' analgesia, omitting those reporting 'fair/slight/poor' (authors' scales vary substantially)

but improved over the four months and yielded a sample of 38 primigravidae and 22 multigravidae. One scalp, one hand and three leg points were used, on one side of the body only, and manual or electrical stimulation were employed as necessary. Additional analgesia was available, but was needed in the first stage for four primigravidae and one multipara only, whilst Apgar scores of all babies were 8 or above. Particularly impressive are the quoted average induction to delivery times (4 hours 45 mins for primigravidae and 2 hours 30 mins for multigravidae versus 8 hours 30 mins and 3 hours 45 mins in the respective control groups), and the claim that low forceps delivery and manual removal of placenta could usually be carried out under acupuncture alone.

Umeh (1986) utilised a different approach for 30 Nigerian women. She sited long acupuncture needles subcutaneously and parallel to the skin on either side of the sacrum, so that the handles and points protruded, then manipulated the needles for at least 20 minutes, later padding and taping them in place. Almost two thirds of primiparae and multiparae had vaginal deliveries using acupuncture alone, 20 per cent of the total registering no pain throughout their labour on visual analogue scales completed at 15 minute intervals. The remaining mothers (37 per cent) received pethidine later in labour. No adverse effects on mother or neonate were noted, nor was there any effect on the length of labour. Impressions of mothers and staff were favourable, and the author concludes that, although effectiveness varies, the technique is worth promoting, especially in developing countries where staffing and finances do not permit use of sophisticated analgesic techniques such as epidurals.

Donley (1987) reported the use of acupuncture since 1977 by some domiciliary midwives in New Zealand, not only for analgesia during home births, but also for augmentation of labour, version of breech presentation at about 34 weeks, raised blood pressure, retained placenta, stimulation of poor lactation and to relieve after pains. Such treatment was used for about 13 per cent of the home deliveries in the Auckland area in 1986. The article depicts the acupuncture points used for each condition.

In a report from Sweden (Lyrenäs *et al* 1987a) the authors tested a finding from Germany that acupuncture administered during the last few weeks of pregnancy could shorten labour for primigravidae and possibly raise the pain threshold in subjects prior to delivery. They used acupuncture in this way on 56 primiparous women and found that the length of both pregnancy and labour, especially the second stage, were slightly longer compared with three other groups of nulliparous women. The subjects' personal experience of labour was not recorded but analgesic requirements were similar for all study groups.

These findings should be interpreted with caution, since there were significant variations in length of gestation between the groups. The control group comprised all the adjacent nulliparous women from the delivery suite register, some of whom had delivered prematurely, and the two smaller reference groups were women who registered after the start of the main study and those who volunteered for lumbar puncture at 38 weeks for a related study. The acupuncture and lumbar puncture groups appear from the figures to have all reached the treatment gestations of 36+ and 38 weeks respectively, hence did not include any premature deliveries. The acupuncture group received weekly treatments from 36 weeks until delivery; inevitably one would find a positive correlation between length of pregnancy and number of treatments. The findings that the second stage of labour was longer and more operative deliveries were required may also be partially explained by the apparently longer gestations of the acupuncture group.

O'Driscoll's definition of the onset of labour was used (O'Driscoll & Meagher 1986) – that is the arrival of the mother in established labour at the delivery suite ignoring any prior time not confirmable by hospital staff. This is internally consistent but would clearly affect comparison with other studies.

In a companion report, Lyrenäs *et al* (1987b) failed to find any transient or long term effect of this mode of acupuncture on cerebrospinal fluid endorphins, and therefore ruled this out as a mechanism for increasing pain threshold prior to delivery.

Skelton, a research midwife in Glasgow, evaluated electro-acupuncture given to 85 women, with a matched control group receiving conventional analgesia (Skelton & Flowerdew 1988). Entonox was available to all women, and 48 parturients achieved delivery using acupuncture and Entonox. Thirty-five women using acupuncture received further pharmacological analgesics, dubbed 'acupuncture-plus'. Only 10 of these cases were attributed to inadequate analgesia, the rest being very distressed on admission or having complicated labours. Significantly lower pain scores (visual analogue scales) were found for multiparae than nulliparae in all treatment groups, as expected. Multiparae using acupuncture successfully registered lower pain scores than control or acupuncture-plus multiparae, whilst amongst nulliparae scores were significantly worse for the acupuncture-plus group than for controls or successful acupuncture users. Overall, pain scores were lower for women who had attended antenatal classes.

A questionnaire on the third postnatal day revealed that more women receiving acupuncture felt in control of their labour and delivery and were 'very satisfied' with their analgesia. These differences were not influenced by social class, age, anxiety or muscle tension scores. Women receiving pethidine alone (52 mothers) were more likely to report 'little' or 'no' pain relief, whereas those having epidurals reported optimum pain relief. The first stage of labour was significantly shorter (average 2.5 hrs shorter) for nulliparae having acupuncture.

☐ **Acupunture and TENS – a summary**

Whilst there is undoubtedly some overlap in the mechanisms of action of TENS, electro-acupuncture and other forms of acupuncture (Melzack

1984b), the logistics of introducing these differing therapies in a maternity unit merits consideration.

As observed in many articles, acupuncture should not be viewed primarily as analgesia for labour, but as potential treatment for such pregnancy related conditions as back pain, vomiting and other digestive disorders, migraine, raised blood pressure, malpresentations and for induction of labour and insufficient lactation (Skelton & Flowerdew 1985). TENS also has a variety of applications, but mostly these are aimed at relief of painful perinatal conditions for the mother. TENS availability and training have already been discussed.

Arranging acupuncture for labour may be daunting, as the practitioner would have to be 'on call'. A private therapist may be expensive, whilst the few NHS midwives qualified in acupuncture may have workloads that prevent them from guaranteeing their availability for specific women in labour. Hence unless there are enough specialised staff to provide a viable service, the option of acupuncture may not be offered to potential clients, unless they specifically ask. Such issues are confronted in an article by Boxx (1984) addressed to fellow practitioners and stressing that obstetric acupuncture should only be attempted by those competent in both disciplines.

Of the 30 or so acupuncture points relevant to the location of labour pain, a number are located on the back, abdomen or even perineum, and are not, therefore, likely to be valuable to a mobile woman throughout labour. Points on the limbs, or auriculo-acupuncture are generally recommended instead. The latter may be effected by the use of 'presspins' which, once positioned in the outer ear, may be manipulated by the mother herself during contractions. Acupuncture can be used alone or with supplementary analgesia if required, and there are no contraindications to its use in women at term (Skelton & Flowerdew 1985).

Neither acupuncture nor TENS rely on previous practice on the part of the mother, unlike hypnosis. TENS requires more expensive equipment but acupuncture requires more specific staff training, only available from external agencies. Both techniques have wider uses than labour analgesia but, on balance, a TENS service is probably more easily introduced for most maternity services.

□ **Homoeopathy**

Homoeopathy was developed single handedly by Dr Samuel Hahnemann early in the last century and is the antithesis of conventional allopathic medicine. The basic tenet is that 'like cures like', thus for a fever, instead of giving an antipyretic, one would give a dilute natural substance which was capable of causing fever at a higher concentration. The aim is to fortify the body's own reaction to the fever, rather than to antagonise or suppress it.

Homoeopathic remedies are prepared from plant or mineral sources, some of which are common to herbalism, and many have been the subject of research by pharmaceutical companies seeking to confirm and purify the active ingredients. The remedies are obtained by an elaborate process of dilution in stages, resulting in solutions, ointments or tablets which theoretically would contain only a few molecules of the active substance. The most dilute are held to have the most potent effect in the body, with the decreasing concentrations being referred to as 6X, 12X, 30X etc. They may be obtained from many health or wholefood shops without a prescription, but there are also many medically qualified doctors who practise homoeopathy, either solely or in conjunction with orthodox 'allopathic' medicine. During pregnancy professional advice, rather than self-medication, is well advised. As with other holistic systems, a practitioner will consider the individual client's overall physical and psychological state, rather than prescribing on the basis of a single symptom or disease.

Remedies are available for such pregnancy disorders as nausea, constipation and haemorrhoids, also as toning agents for the uterus to promote an easier labour, for example caulophyllum (blue cohosh or squaw root). This latter remedy can also be used to augment labour and to forestall haemorrhage. Arnica (from an alpine flower) can be valuable before, during and after labour to relieve pain and bruising (Junor & Monaco 1984). Remedies also exist for painful breasts and insufficient lactation.

☐ Herbs and flowers

Herbalism has a long history, and many herbs contain high concentrations of useful vitamins and minerals. Again, there are trained practitioners of herbal medicine (or naturopathy) and a number of specialist shops and books. Remedies are obtainable without a prescription. Certain herbs should be avoided throughout pregnancy, and others should only be used during the last month, to prepare the body for the birth process, so it is essential to get authoritative advice. A useful precis of herbs applicable in midwifery is given by Bunce (1987). Summaries for prospective users may be found (Junor and Monaco 1984; Claxton and Rudd 1986). Herbal remedies are usually prepared, from fresh or dried plants, by infusing a small amount of the root or leaves in hot water, then drinking as a 'tea'. Increasingly, tablets and capsules are also becoming available.

A variety of herbal remedies exist for early pregnancy sickness, high blood pressure, constipation, problems with lactation and perineal discomfort. Preparations for sore nipples containing chamomile or marigold (calendula) are gaining 'mainstream' popularity.

Probably the most widely known herb for use in pregnancy is raspberry leaf, rich in iron and vitamin C, and used to tonify the uterus during the last few months of pregnancy so as to promote an easier labour. Raspberry leaf is also a component of herbal mixtures for use during pregnancy, and a formula for use during labour to help stimulate effective contractions.

Another mixture, used by many homoeopaths and independent midwives, is Rescue Remedy, containing the extracts of five flowers, which can be used in small quantities throughout labour to alleviate panic, shock and detachment from reality. It is one of several dozen flower remedies developed by Dr Edward Bach earlier this century, his philosophy being that physical illness and pain are exacerbated by stress and negative attitudes, and that certain flower extracts can flood the body with positive and beautiful vibrations to counter disease (Junor & Monaco 1984).

☐ **Massage techniques**

Reflexology, or reflex zone therapy, refers to massage of specific parts of the body, especially the soles of the feet, in order to influence distant areas (Lett 1983). The sole is considered to have points on its surface which relate to all other organs of the body (similar to the role of the ear in auriculotherapy). Massage of these points induces wellbeing, and there are several techniques used to reduce labour pain (Sakala 1988). Related research is lacking, and its use in midwifery (at least in Britain) is rare.

Another technique, *effleurage* (meaning 'feather touch') is essentially light abdominal massage. This is done in rhythmic stroking patterns over the lower abdomen with the pads of the fingers, enhanced by the use of talcum powder. An attendant or partner can do this by gently drawing alternate hands across the lower abdomen from one side to the other. The woman herself can use a similar pattern with one hand then the other, tracing below her 'bump', or can use both hands, with fingers slightly separated, to stroke lightly down the centre of the abdomen and up the lateral areas (or vice versa), thus describing two large circles (Varney 1980). Some women find this very comforting, and a good distraction if they are performing it themselves, others dislike any touching of the abdomen.

Heat and cold can also be used to beneficial effect. Many women gain great comfort from heat (for example, in the form of hot towels) against their back or lower abdomen, and a few benefit from cold compresses to painful areas. In fact the use of alternating hot and cold compresses is most sound physiologically, as this avoids the area becoming ischaemic.

Back-rubbing is a very relaxing and effective procedure for many; apart from generalised massage over the back, shoulders or thighs with talcum powder or oil, a technique referred to in Varney (1980) as the OB back rub is essential for any midwife or labour partner to learn. It consists of steady deep kneading over the lower spine, with the aim being to move the palm of the attendant and the skin of the mother as one over the underlying tissues. This is done in slow small circles, without creating friction actually on the mother's skin. It is usually most helpful during contractions, and the attendant can counter fatigue by bracing his or her arm against the body or bed, in order to apply the right degree of pressure over a prolonged period.

Further possibilities which may appeal to motivated women are the use of *nipple stimulation* or *clitoral massage* by the woman herself or her partner: either technique may alleviate pain but they are primarily suggested to augment contractions in a slow labour, possibly enabling a woman to manage without further analgesia (Gaskin 1980; Gillie 1986; Smith 1986).

☐ **Hypnosis**

Hypnosis is defined as 'a temporarily altered state of consciousness in which the individual has increased suggestibility' (Vadurro & Butts 1982). Its use in medicine and dentistry has been documented from 1821 onwards, the two major applications being in psychotherapy and in hypno-analgesia/ anaesthesia. Often thought of as a 'fringe' technique, and sought only as a last resort for intractable and inadequately understood pain such as migraine headaches, hypnosis is actually more successful when used for acute organically-based pain. In good subjects its success is well above the placebo level, and in studies where humans have been subjected to pain experimentally, hypnosis has been reported to be more effective than morphine, aspirin, diazepam or acupuncture (Orne & Dinges 1984). Hypnosis is rarely offered by maternity units in Britain, but is occasionally available from hospital medical staff, GPs (a few medical schools include it in their syllabus), psychotherapists or indeed midwives trained in its use.

It has been found that individuals have different levels of suggestibility, and that the hypnotic response may be easily inhibited by the subject if conditions are not favourable. The subject's hypnotisability can be deter- mined at an early stage by the use of the Stanford Hypnotic Susceptibility Scale (Weitzenhoffer & Hilgard 1967). Estimates of the number of people who would be good subjects for hypno-anaesthesia for operations vary from less than 10 per cent to over 90 per cent according to the type of surgery to be undergone. Additionally, many subjects who do not achieve marked pain relief from hypnosis will still benefit from the practice of relaxation and reduction of anxiety.

Doubts are raised by authors such as Hearne (1986), whose concern hinges around hypnosis in front of an audience, and the tendency of subjects under stress to comply with expectations. In modern practice, the image of the helpless subject being 'dominated' has been replaced by emphasis on a partnership between therapist and subject.

There are three stages for successful hypnosis: the hypnotisability of the client, the establishment of rapport, and the actual procedure of hypnosis (which can be divided into hypnotic induction and subsequent suggestion of pain relief).

Hypnotic induction may take many forms, common ones being focused attention on the therapist's voice (speaking in a monotone), in conjunction with either eye fixation on an object on the other side of the room, or watching a pendulum or a moving hand. The subject may be 'counted down' to deeper levels of trance, and is later returned to full consciousness by further counting.

Examples of specific suggestion techniques for analgesia under hypnosis are outlined by Orne and Dinges (1984). Three possible approaches are: to imagine the painful area going numb and heavy, via pins and needles to a sensation of deadness (as after administration of a local anaesthetic); to imagine the affected limb or organ floating outside the body, so that the pain is also targetted outside the body; or to focus the pain into one's clenched fist, then throw it away. Suggestion can also be given to enhance the subject's self esteem, ability to sleep and feeling of wellbeing, also to rehearse the stages of labour.

Whilst the pain is relieved, pressure and touch sensations are still perceived, also the autonomic reactions to the painful stimulus will continue. A labouring woman using hypnosis is not detached from her surroundings, as in sleep, but can remain alert to her progress, move freely and converse with her attendants, although during contractions she will need her full concentration, with eyes closed and minimal extraneous noises.

It is possible for a woman to be taught to induce self-hypnosis, or for her partner to provide the inductive stimulus, such as stroking her hand, so that hypnosis can be used at will. Ideally, training sessions for individuals or small groups should start early in the second trimester and continue, eventually weekly, until term.

□   **Research into the use of hypnosis**

Case studies of highly successful births under hypnosis are given by Gartside (1982) and Vadurro and Butts (1982). There is also documented evidence of hypnosis as the sole method of analgesia for caesarean section, hysterectomy and as psychotherapy for severe nausea in early pregnancy (Orne & Dinges 1984). Descriptions of hypnosis techniques for use in childbirth can be found in August (1961), Scott (1974), Kroger (1977) and Stone and Burrows (1980).

Trials of hypnosis in labour have not involved large numbers of women, nor have they usually been randomised. Freeman *et al* (1986) tested a previous claim that labour under self-hypnosis was shorter and analgesia enhanced. Eighty-two nulliparae were randomly allocated to a hypnosis group or a control group, all attending routine antenatal classes. The experimental group were also attending hypnosis sessions, on an individual basis, from 32 weeks of pregnancy. Four women failed to attend for hypnosis and 13 were excluded because of obstetric complications.

Ultimately 29 women used self-hypnosis in labour; five of these were assessed antenatally as good hypnotic subjects, nineteen as moderate and five as poor. No significant differences were found in efficacy of pain relief, the actual use of other analgesia or in the mode of delivery. An unexpected result was that the mean duration of both pregnancy and labour were longer in the hypnosis group, although these womens' satisfaction with labour was also higher. There is no information, however, as to whether all the women had spontaneous labours, nor as to how the length of labour was assessed.

Brann & Guzvica (1987), working in an English general practice, introduced the option of self-hypnosis versus psychoprophylaxis to expectant mothers of any parity. Hypnosis sessions were supplemented with a cassette tape for home practice, with the reverse side for use in labour, both involving visualisation of a beach scene, with the sound of waves appearing on the tape behind the voice. The 45 clients using self-hypnosis had shorter labours than the psychoprophylaxis group, higher satisfaction scores and lower use of other analgesics, despite the former comprising more nulliparae and having a higher average age. The authors considered some additional criteria such as Apgar scores, and success at breastfeeding, where no differences were displayed. They mention that other more 'successful' authors reported studies in which the hypnotist was present during labour, whereas their own endeavour was to provide a valid comparison with psychoprophylaxis, where the tutor would not usually be present during labour. They also conclude that to achieve a reduction in labour time, specific suggestion to this effect is necessary during training.

□ **Sophrology**

A related technique is sophrology, popularised in France and Spain in the past 30 years, and described in a French childbirth magazine as 'at the crossroads of relaxation, yoga, hypnosis and auto-suggestion' (Planiol 1988). The term seems to have been devised as an alternative to hypnosis, to dispel any negative associations of the latter (Berland *et al* 1988).

Preparation may be as individuals or in groups, with voice/music tapes to listen to. The mother focuses on her breathing, on visualising effective contractions of the uterus and relaxation of the cervix and perineum – in short, an increased body awareness, whilst in a state of 'hypo-vigilance' (Leroy 1987). A woman may train to experience each contraction as a pleasant warmth, rather than as pain. Sophrology has found other applications in improving professional sports (such as skiing) performances, through prior mental visualisation of an ideal performance, and elimination of nervousness and fatigue (Ostrander *et al* 1981).

There is conflicting evidence about the benefits of hypnosis and sophrology in obstetrics. The techniques require a high degree of motivation and invested time, but have no reported side effects on mother or baby, and deserve further evaluation by larger-scale studies.

To conclude this chapter, readers are encouraged to evaluate their approach to pain relief in labour by considering the following recommendations and practice checklist.

■ Recommendations for clinical practice in the light of currently available evidence

It is recommended that midwives should:

1 Administer pethidine only when labour is established.

2 Consider the use of naloxone to reverse neonatal respiratory depression induced by narcotic analgesia such as pethidine.

3 Ensure that they are competent in epidural 'top-up' technique.

4 Review the timing of pushing in cases where the client has just received an epidural 'top-up' in the second stage of labour.

5 Give clear explanation to women before an epidural is sited and give emotional support so that these women do not feel like 'failures'.

6 Give clear instruction to clients receiving inhalation analgesia via the Entonox machine.

7 Seek information on local practitioners of alternative therapies, especially acupuncturists and homoeopathic doctors, in order that they can offer prospective mothers information or contacts for the full range of therapies.

8 Always endeavour to support the mother in her choice of analgesia, and ensure that this is an informed choice.

9 Be taught how to administer TENS, and increase their collaborations with obstetric physiotherapists who are experienced in the use of the technique.

10 Support more research on the long and short term outcomes for mother and baby of the alternative therapies discussed, in order to establish their value and freedom from side effects.

■ Practice check

● Is there a policy regarding types and amount of analgesia administered by midwives in your unit? If yes, how often is this policy updated?

- Is there a planned programme of in-service training for epidural top-ups?

- Do you evaluate the effectiveness of different forms of analgesia used for women in labour – for example by using the verbal or visual analogue scales described in this chapter?

- Do you evaluate the client's satisfaction regarding analgesia administered during labour?

- Is there a forum in your unit whereby midwives and doctors can discuss the above issues?

■ References

Abboud T K, Afrasiabi A, Sarkis F, Daftarian F, Nagappala S, Noueihed R, Kuhnert B, Miller F 1984a Continuous infusion epidural analgesia in parturients receiving bupivacaine, chloroprocaine, or lidocaine – maternal fetal and neonatal effects. Anesthesia and Analgesia 63: 421–28

Abboud T K, Shnider S M, Dailey P A, Raya J A, Sarkis F, Grobler N M, Sadri S, Khoo S S, Desousa B, Baysinger O L, Miller F 1984b Intrathecal administration of hyperbaric morphine for the relief of pain in labour. British Journal of Anaesthesia 56: 1351–58

Abouleish E, Depp R 1975 Acupuncture in obstetrics. Anesthesia and Analgesia 54(1): 82–8

Ackerman W E, Colclough G W 1987 Prophylactic epidural blood patch: the controversy continues. Anesthesia and Analgesia 60: 913

August R V 1961 Hypnosis in obstetrics. McGraw-Hill, New York

Augustinsson L-E, Bohlin P, Bundsen P, Carlsson C-A, Forssman L, Sjoberg P, Tyreman N O 1977 Pain relief during delivery by transcutaneous electrical nerve stimulation. Pain 4: 59–65

Bates R G, Helm O W, Duncan A, Edmonds D K 1985 Uterine activity in the second stage of labour and the effect of epidural analgesia. British Journal of Obstetrics and Gynaecology 92(12): 1246–50

Baxter K G 1983 Transcutaneous nerve stimulation: efficacy of clinical applications. Journal of the Kansas Medical Society 84(1): 18–26; 38

Belsey E M, Rosenblatt D B, Lieberman B A, Redshaw M, Caldwell J, Notarianni L, Smith R L, Beard R W 1981 The influence of maternal analgesia on neonatal behaviour: 1 pethidine. British Journal of Obstetrics and Gynaecology 88: 398–406

Bendiner E 1985 Medicine in China – validating the venerable and investigating the new. Hospital Practice 20(6): 37–44

Berland M, Miellet C, Monnet F, Irrmann M, Marsaud H, Broussalian G, Broussard P 1988 La verité sur les methodes non invasives d'analgesie obstetricale: Table Ronde Des Journees Lyonnaises. (Round Table: The truth about non-invasive methods of obstetric analgesia). Revue Française de Gynecologie et d'Obstetrique 83(2): 75–84

Bogod D G, Rosen M, Rees G A D 1987 Extradural infusion of 0.125% bupivacaine at 10ml H–1 to women during labour. British Journal of Anaesthesia 59: 325–30

Bonica J J 1984 Labour pain. In Wall P D and Melzack R (eds) Textbook of pain. Churchill Livingstone, London

Bonica J J, Akamatsu T J, Berges P U, Morikawa K, Kennedy W F (1971) Circulatory effects of peridural block II: effects of epinephrine. Anaesthesiology 34: 514–22

Bonta B W, Gagliardi J V, Williams V, Warshaw J B 1979 Naloxone reversal of mild neurobehavioural depression in normal newborn infants after routine obstetric analgesia. Journal of paediatrics 94(1): 102–5

Box D 1984 Made in Japan. Nursing Times 80(17): 39–40

Boxx P J 1984 Acupuncture in childbirth. British Journal of Acupuncture 7(1): 22–4

Brahams D 1982 Record award for personal injuries sustained as a result of negligent administration of epidural anaesthetic. Lancet i: 159

Brann L R, Guzvica S A 1987 Comparison of hypnosis with conventional relaxation for antenatal and intrapartum use: a feasability study in general practice. Journal of the Royal College of General Practitioners 37(3): 437–40

Brazelton T B 1973 Neonatal behavioural assessment scale. Spastics Medical Press, London

British Medical Association 1984 The uses of acupuncture: evidence from the British Medical Acupuncture Society. BMA News Review 10(7): 15–16

Bunce K L 1987 The use of herbs in midwifery. Journal of Nurse–Midwifery 32(4): 255–9. Reproduced in MIDIRS Pack 7, April 1988

Bundsen P 1982 Pain relief in labour. Acta Obstetrica et Gynecologica Scandinavica 61: 289–97

Bundsen P, Ericson K 1982 Pain relief in labor by transcutaneous electrical nerve stimulation: safety aspects. Acta Obstetrica et Gynecologica Scandinavica 61: 1–5

Bundsen P, Ericson K, Peterson L-E, Thiringer K 1982 Pain relief in labor by transcutaneous electrical nerve stimulation. Acta Obstetrica et Gynecologica Scandinavica 61: 129–36

Bundsen P, Peterson L-E, Selstam U 1981 Pain relief in labor by transcutaneous electrical nerve stimulation: a prospective matched study. Acta Obstetrica et Gynecologica Scandinavica 60: 459–68

Buxton E J, Redman C W E, Obhrai M 1988 Delayed pushing with lumbar epidural in labour – does it increase the incidence of spontaneous delivery? Journal of Obstetrics and Gynaecology 8: 258–61

Carrie I E S, O'Sullivan G M, Leegobin R 1981 Epidural fentanyl in labour. Anaesthesia 36: 965–69

Celleno D, Capogna G 1988 Epidural fentanyl plus bupivacaine 0.125% for labour: analgesic effects. Canadian Anesthesiology 35(4): 375–8

Chapman O R 1977 Sensory decision theory methods in pain research. Pain 3: 295–305

Cheek T G, Banner R, Sater J, Gutsche B B 1988 Prophylactic extradural blood patch. British Journal of Anaesthesia 61: 340–42

Chestnut D H, Owen C L, Bates J N, Ostman L G, Choi W W, Geiger M E 1988 Continuous infusion epidural analgesia during labour: a randomised, double-blind comparison of 0.0625% bupivacaine /0.0002% fentanyl versus 0.125% bupivacaine. Anesthesiology 68: 754–59

Chestnut D H, Vandewalker G E, Owen O L, Bates J N, Choi W W 1987 The influence of continuous epidural bupivacaine analgesia on the second stage of labour and method of delivery on the nulliparous woman. Anesthesiology 66: 774–80

Claxton R, Rudd C 1986 Natural healing – a holistic approach to health. In Claxton R (ed) Birth matters: issues and alternatives in childbirth. Unwin, London

Crawford J S 1982 The effect of epidural block on the progress of labour. In Studd J (ed) Progress in obstetrics and gynaecology, Vol 2. Churchill Livingstone, Edinburgh

Crawford J S 1986 Some maternal complications of epidural analgesia for labour. Obstetric Anaesthesia Digest 6(2): 221–22

Crawford J S, Davies P, Pearson J F 1973 Significance of the individual components of the Apgar score. British Journal of Anaesthesia 45: 148

DHSS 1987 Safety information bulletin SIB(87) 23: Fetal monitors: interference of fetal heart rate traces caused by the use of transcutaneous electrical nerve stimulation equipment during labour. HMSO, London

Dorman F M, Wright J T 1983 A prospective study on the second stage of labour following epidural analgesia. Journal of Obstetrics and Gynaecology 4: 40–1

Donley J 1987 Acupuncture: an alternative method of pain relief. Article From New Zealand Midwives' Seminar, June 1987. Reprinted in MIDIRS Information Pack 7, April 1988

Dutton D A, Moir D D, Howie H B, Thorburn J, Watson R 1984 Choice of local anaesthetic drug for extradural caesarean section. British Journal of Anaesthesia 56(12): 1361–68

Faure B A M, Bart A J, Koht A 1980 A comparison of continuous infusion epidural analgesia versus intermittent injection technique for obstetrical pain relief. Anesthesiology 53: S294

Feely J, Williams G R, McAllister O B, Wood A J J 1982 Increased toxicity and reduced clearance of lidocaine by cimetidine. Annals of Internal Medicine 96: 592

Flynn A M, Kelly J, Hollins G, Lynch P F 1978 Ambulation in labour. British Medical Journal 2: 591–93

Flynn R J, Moore J, Collier P S, McClean E 1989 Does pretreatment with cimetidine and ranitidine affect the disposition of bupivacaine? British Journal of Anaesthesia 62: 87–91

Fordyce W E 1973 An operant conditioning method for managing pain. Postgraduate Medicine 53: 123

Frank M, Heywood A, Macleod D M 1988 Survey of the practice of epidural analgesia in a regional sample of obstetric units. Anaesthesia 43: 54–8

Freeman R M, Macaulay A J, Eve L, Chamberlain G V P, Bhat A V 1986 Randomised trial of self hypnosis for analgesia in labour. British Medical Journal 292: 657–58

Gaskin I M 1980 Spiritual midwifery, revised ed. The Book Publishing Company, Summertown, Tennessee

Gartside G 1982 Easy labour – a personal experience of childbirth under hypnosis. Nursing Times 78(51): 2187–88

Gillie O 1986 A tweak to ease labour pains. The Independent 9 December, Reprinted in MIDIRS pack 3, December 1986

Goodfellow C F, Hull M G R 1983 Oxytocin deficiency at delivery with epidural analgesia. British Journal of Obstetrics and Gynaecology 90: 214–19

Goodman L S, Gilman A 1965 The pharmacological basis of therapeutics, 3rd ed. New York, Macmillan

Gottschalk W, Hamilton L A 1975 Paracervical-pudendal blocks in obstetrics. Clinics in Obstetrics and Gynaecology 2(3): 565–77

Gowers S R 1985 A stimulating experience. Midwives Chronicle 98(1174): 295–96

Grim L C, Morey S H 1985 Transcutaneous electrical nerve stimulation for relief of parturition pain: a clinical report. Physical Therapy 65(3): 337–40

Harrison R F, Woods T, Shore M, Mathews G, Unwin A 1986 Pain relief in labour using transcutaneous electrical nerve stimulation (TENS): a TENS/ TENS placebo controlled study in two parity groups. British Journal of Obstetrics and Gynaecology 93: 739–46

Harrison R F, Shore M, Woods T, Mathews G, Gardiner J, Unwin A 1987 A comparative study of TENS, Entonox, pethidine and promazine and lumbar epidural for pain relief in labour. Acta Obstetrica Gynecologica Scandinavica 66: 9–14

Head H, Rivers W, Sherren J 1905 The afferent nervous system from a new aspect. Brain 28: 99

Hearne K 1986 Hypnosis – is it of value? Pulse 46(21): 77

Heywood A M 1989 Unpublished data

Hibbard B M, Rosen M, Davies D 1986 Placental transfer of naloxone. British Journal of Anaesthesia 58: 45–8

Hodgkinson R, Bhatt M, Wang C N 1978 Double-blind comparison of the neurobehaviour of neonates following the administration of different doses of meperidine to mother. Canadian Anaesthesia Society Journal 25(5): 405–08

Hodgkinson R, Husain F J 1982 The duration of maternally administered meperidine on neonatal neurobehaviour. Anesthesiology 56: 51–2

Holdcroft A, Morgan M 1974 An assessment of the analgesic effect in labour of pethidine and 50 per cent nitrous oxide in oxygen (Entonox). The Journal of Obstetrics and Gynaecology of the British Commonwealth 81: 603–07

Hughes S C, Rosen M A, Shnider S M, Abboud T K, Stefani S J, Norton M 1981 Maternal and neonatal effects of epidural morphine for labour and delivery. Anesthesia Analgesia 63: 319

Husemeyer R P, Davenport H T, Cummings, A J, Rosankiewicz J R 1981 Comparison of epidural and intramuscular pethidine for analgesia in labour. British Journal of Obstetrics and Gynaecology 88(7): 711–17

Hyodo M, Gega O 1977 Use of acupuncture anesthesia for normal delivery. American Journal of Chinese Medicine 5(1): 63–9

Junor V, Monaco M 1984 Home birth handbook: 118–23. Souvenir Press, London

Keenan D L, Simonsen L, McCrann D J 1985 Transcutaneous electrical nerve stimulation for pain control during labour and delivery: a case report. Physical Therapy 9: 1363–64

Kitzinger S 1988 Some women's experiences of epidurals. National Childbirth Trust, London

Knepp N B, Cheer G, Gutshe B B 1983 Bupivacaine: continuous infusion epidural analgesia for labour. Anesthesiology 59: A407

Kroger W S 1977 Clinical and experimental hypnosis, 2nd ed. J B Lippincott, Philadelphia

Kubista E, Kucera H 1976 versuche mit elektro-akupunktur zur analgesie wahrend der geburt. (experiments of electro-acupuncture-analgesia during deliveryy: author's translation.) Geburtshilfe Frauenheilkd 36(7): 610–13

Latham J 1987 Pain control. Lisa Sainsbury Foundation Series. Austen Cornish, Reading

Lett A 1983 Putting their best feet forward. Nursing Times 79(32): 49–51

Leroy M 1987 Intérèt de la preparation a l'accouchement. Soins Gynecologiques, Obstetriques, Pueriques et Pediatriques 78: 37–41

Levinson G, Shnider S M, de Lorimier A, Steffenson J L 1974 Effects of maternal hyperventilation on uterine blood flow and fetal oxygenation and acid-base status. Anesthesiology 40(4): 340–46

Lewith G T 1982 Acupuncture: its place in western medical science: 43–8. Thorsons, Wellingborough

Lindblad A, Bernow J, Marsal K 1987 Obstetric analgesia and fetal aortic blood flow during labour. British Journal of Obstetrics and Gynaecology 94: 306–11

Livingston W K 1943 Pain mechanisms: a physiologic interpretation of causalgia and its related states. Macmillan, New York

Loeser E A, Hill G E, Bennet G M, Sederbay J H 1978 Time versus success rate for epidural bupivacaine. Anesthesiology 49: 147–48

Lowe N K 1987 Individual variation in childbirth pain. Journal of Psychosomatic obstetrics and Gynaecology 7(3): 183–92

Lyrenäs S, Lutsch H, Hetta J, Lindberg B 1987a Acupuncture before delivery: effect on labour. Gynecologic and Obstetric Investigation 24: 217–24

Lyrenäs S, Nyberg F, Lutsch H, Lindberg B, Terenius L 1987b Cerebrospinal fluid dynorphin$_{1-17}$ and β-endorphin in late pregnancy and six months after delivery. No influence of acupuncture treatment. Acta Endocrinologica (Copenhagen) 115: 253–58

Lyons G, MacDonald R 1985 Difficult intubation in obstetrics. Anesthesiology 40: 1016

Maresh M, Choong K H, Beard R W 1983 Delayed pushing with lumbar epidural analgesia in labour. British Journal of Obstetrics and Gynaecology 90: 623–27

Meiyu S 1985 Acupuncture anaesthesia for caesarean section. Midwives Chronicle 98(1167): 107

Melzack R, Wall P D 1965 Pain mechanisms: a new theory. Science 150: 971–79

Melzack R 1984a, Measurement of the dimension of pain experience. In Bromm B (ed) Pain measurement in man: neurophysiological correlates of pain. Elsevier, Amsterdam

Melzack R 1984b Acupuncture and other related forms of folk medicine. In Wall P D Melzack R (eds) Textbook of pain. Churchill Livingstone, London

Mendez-Bauer C J 1980 A perspective of maternal position during labour. Journal of Perinatal Medicine 8: 255–64

Merry A F 1983 Use of transcutaneous electrical nerve stimulation in labour. New Zealand Medical Journal   August 10: 635–36

Milner I 1988 Water baths for pain relief in labour. Nursing Times   84(1): 39–40. Reproduced in MIDIRS Pack 8, August 1988

Mitchell M, Harris A, Mullinger B M 1987 Ranitidine drug interactions – a literature review. Pharmocology and Therapeutics   32: 293–325

Moir D D 1970 Increased anaesthesia for caesarean section: an evaluation of a method being low concentrations of halothane and 50% oxygen. British Journal of Anaesthesia   42: 136–42

Moir D D 1986 Obstetric anaesthesia and analgesia, 5th ed. Baillière Tindall, London

Morgan B M 1982a Double-blind comparison of meptazinol and pethidine in labour. British Journal of Obstetrics and Gynaecology   89: 318–22

Morgan B M, Bulpitt C J, Clifton P, Lewis P J 1982b Analgesia and satisfaction in childbirth (the Queen Charlotte's 1000 mother survey). Lancet   ii: 808–10

Mowat J, Garrey M M 1970 Comparison of pentazocine and pethidine in labour. British Medical Journal 2: 757

Munley A J, Railton R, Gray W M, Carter K B 1986 Exposure of midwives to nitrous oxide in 4 hospitals. British Medical Journal   258: 1063–64

Murray A D, Dolby R M, Nation R L, Thomas D B 1981 Effects of epidural anaesthesia on newborns and their mothers. Child Development   52(1): 71–82

Nicholas A D G, Robson P J 1982 Double-blind comparison of meptazinol and pethidine in labour. British Journal of Obstetrics and Gynaecology   89: 318–22

Niv D, Ruddick V, Golan A, Chayen M S 1986 Augmentation of bupivacaine analgesia in labour by epidural morphine. Obstetrics and Gynaecology   67: 206

Nybell-Lindahl G, Carlsoan C 1981 Maternal and fetal concentrations of morphine after epidural administration during labour. American Journal of Obstetrics and Gynecology   139: 20

Oakley A 1980 Women confined. Martin Robertson, Oxford

O'Driscoll K, Meagher D 1986 Active management of labour – the Dublin experience, 2nd ed. Balliere Tindall, London

Ogbonna B, Daw E 1986 Epidural analgesia and the length of labour for vaginal twin delivery. Journal of Obstetrics and Gynaecology   6: 166–68

Orne M T Dinges D F 1984 Hypnosis. In Wall P D Melzack R D (ed) Textbook of pain. Churchill Livingstone, London

Osler M 1987 A double-blind study comparing meptazinol and pethidine for pain relief in labour. European Journal of Obstetrics and Gynaecology   26: 15–18

Ostrander S, Schroeder L, Ostrander N 1981 Superlearning. Sphere, London

Perera W S E 1979 Acupuncture in childbirth. British Journal of Acupuncture   2(1): 12–14

Pickles S 1987 TNS – a user's view. Association of Chartered Physiotherapists in Obstetrics and Gynaecology Journal   61 (July): 20–2

Planiol F 1988 Toutes les methodes pour accoucher sans douleur. Parents – Hors Serie   Printemps: 64–7

Polden M 1984 Transcutaneous nerve stimulation used in labour. Association of Chartered Physiotherapists in Obstetrics and Gynaecology Journal   54: (Jan) 13–15

Polden M 1985 Transcutaneous nerve stimulation in labour and post-caesarean section. Physiotherapy 71 (7): 350–53

Purdy G, Currie J, Owen H 1987 Continuous extradural analgesics in labour: comparisons between 'on demand' and regular 'top-up' injections. British Journal of Anaesthesia 59(63): 319–24

Read M D, Hunt L P, Anderton J M, Lieberman B A 1983 Psychological aspects of pregnancy. Longman, London

Reid J N, Thorburn J 1988 Extradural bupivacaine or lignocaine anaesthesia for elective caesarean section: the role of maternal posture. British Journal of Anaesthesia 61: 149–53

Reynolds F 1986 Anaesthesia for caesarean section: no more nightmares. Anesthesiology 41: 652

Riffel H D, Nochimson D J, Paul R H, Hon E N G 1973 Effects of meperidine and promethazine during labour. Obstetrics and Gynaecology 42: 738

Robson J E 1979 Transcutaneous nerve stimulation for relief of pain in labour. Anaesthesia 34: 357–60

Rosen M 1977 Pain and its relief. In Chard T, Richards M (eds) Benefits and hazards of the new obstetrics. Heinemann, London

Rosenblatt D B, Belsey E M, Lieberman B A, Redshaw M, Cladwell J, Notarianni L, Beard R W 1981 The influence of maternal analgesia on neonatal behaviour II: epidural bupivacaine. British Journal of Obstetrics and Gynaecology 88: 407–13

Sakala C 1988 Content of care by independent midwives: assistance with pain in labor and birth. Social Science and Medicine 26(11): 1141–58

Salar G, Job I, Mingrino S, Bosio A, Trabucchi M 1981 Effect of transcutaneous electrotherapy of CSF β-endorphin content in patients without pain problems. Pain 10: 169–72

Scott D L 1974 Modern hospital hypnosis: 93–9. Lloyd-Luke, London

Sheikh A, Tunstall M E 1986 Comparative study of meptazinol and pethidine for the relief of pain in labour. British Journal of Obstetrics and Gynaecology 93: 264–9

Shnider S M, Moya F 1974 The anesthesiologist, mother and newborn. Williams and Wilkins, Baltimore

Skelton I, Flowerdew M W 1985 Midwifery and acupuncture. Midwives Chronicle 98(1165): 125–29

Skelton I, Flowerdew M W 1988 Acupuncture and labour. Midwives Chronicle 101(1022): 134–37

Skrabanek P 1984 Acupuncture and the age of unreason. Lancet i: 1169–71

Smith P 1986 Clitoral massage helps ease the pain of labour. She (September): reprinted in MIDIRS pack 3 (December 1986)

Sternbach R A 1974 Pain: patients, traits and treatment: 4. Academic Press, New York:

Stewart P 1979 Transcutaneous nerve stimulation as a method of analgesia in labour. Anaesthesia 34: 361–64

Stewart S 1986 Drug-free pain relief in labour. Nursing Times 82(42): 49–50

Stone P, Burrows G D 1980 Hypnosis and obstetrics. In Burrows G D, Dennerstein L (eds) Handbook of hypnosis and psychosomatic medicine Elsevier, North Holland

Studd J W W, Duigan N D, Crawford J S, Rowbottom C J F, Hughes A 1982 The effect of epidural analgesia on the progress and outcome of induced labour. Journal of Obstetrics and Gynaecology 2: 230–34

Tawfik O, Badraoui M H H, El-Ridi F S 1982 The value of transcutaneous nerve stimulation (TNS) during labour in Egyptian mothers. Schmerz 2: 98–105

Tomkinson J. Turnbull A, Robson G, Dawson I, Cloake E, Adlestein A M, Ashley J E 1982 Report on confidential enquiries into maternal deaths in England and Wales for 1976–79. HMSO, London

Umeh B U O 1986 Sacral acupuncture for pain relief in labour: initial clinical experience in Nigerian women. Acupuncture and Electro-therapeutics Research, International Journal 11: 147–51

United Kingdom Central Council 1986a Handbook of midwives rules. HMSO London

United Kingdom Central Council 1986b Information circular PS&D/86/07: transcutaneous nerve stimulation for the relief of pain in labour. UKCC, London

Vadurro J F, Butts P A 1982 Reducing the anxiety and pain of childbirth through hypnosis. American Journal of Nursing 82(4): 620–23

Vallette C, Niboyet J E, Hebrard M J Favre G 1976 L'analgesie acupuncturale dans l'accouchement. Étude preliminaire. Journal of Gynecology, Obstetrics and Biological Reproduction 5(1): 123–27

Van Zundert A, Vanderaa P P, Van der Donck A, Meeuwis H, Vaes L 1984 Motor blockade expulsion times and instrumental deliveries associated with epidural analgesia for vaginal delivery. Obstetric Anaesthesia Digest 4: 152–56

Varney H 1980 Nurse-midwifery: 204–5. Blackwell Scientific, Boston

Von Frey M 1894 Die gefuhle und ihr verhaltnis zu den empfindungen. Beit z physiol des schmerzsinnes. Berichte uber die verhaltung der konigl sachs. Gesellschaft der Wissenschaften, Leipzig

Wallenstein S L 1984 Scaling clinical pain and pain relief. In Bromm B (ed) Pain measurement in man: neurophysiological correlates of pain: 389–96. Elsevier, Amsterdam

Weddell G 1955 Synthesis and the chemical senses. Annual Review of Psychology 6: 119–36

Weig M 1984 An independent streak. Nursing Times 80(4): 16–8

Weitzenhoffer A M, Hilgard E R 1967 Revised Stanford Profile scales of hypnotic susceptibility. Forms A and B. Consulting Psychologists Press, Palo Alto, CA

Welles B, Belfrage P, de Chateau P 1984 Effects of naloxone on newborn infant behaviour after maternal analgesia with pethidine during labour. Acta Obstetrica Gynecologica Scandinavica 63: 617–19

Werle E 1972 On endogenous producing substances with particular reference to plasmakinins. In Janzen R, Keidel W D, Herz A, Steichele C, Payne J P, Burt R A P (eds) Pain. William and Wilkins, Baltimore

Wilson M C, Spiegelhalter D, Robertson S A, Lesser P 1988 Predicting difficult intubation. British Journal of Anaesthesia 61: 211–16

Woolf C J 1984 Transcutaneous and implanted nerve stimulation. In Wall P D, Melzack R (eds) Textbook of pain. Churchill Livingstone, London

Youngstrom P, Eastwood D, Patel H, Bhatia R, Cowan R, Sutheimeer C 1984 Epidural fentanyl and bupiracaine in labour: double-blind study. Anesthesiology 61: A414

■ Suggested further reading

Avard D M, Nimrod C M 1987 Risks and benefits of obstetric epidural analgesia: a review. Birth   12(4): 215–25

Baxi L, Petrie E 1987 Pharmacologic effects on labour: effects of drugs on dystocia, labour and uterine activity. Clinical Obstetrics and Gynecology 30(1): 19–31

Bevis R 1984 Anaesthesia in midwifery. Baillière Tindall, London

Burt R A P 1971 The fetal and maternal pharmacology of some of the drugs used for the relief of pain in labour. British Journal of Anaesthesia   43: 824–36

Kuhnert B R, Linn P L, Kuhnert P M 1985 Obstetric medication and neonatal behaviour: current controversies. Clinics in Perinatology   12(2): 423–41

McIntyre A 1988 Herbs for pregnancy and childbirth. Sheldon Press, London

Shnider S M, Moya F 1974 The anesthesiologist, mother and newborn. Williams and Wilkins, Baltimore

Sjolund B, Eriksson M 1980 Relief of pain by TENS, English ed. John Wiley, Chichester

Sofaer B 1984 Pain: a handbook for nurses. Harper and Row, London

Tiran M D 1988 Complementary medicine and midwifery. Midwives Chronicle   101(1022): 139–42

■ Useful contacts for non-pharmacological methods

This list is given as a selection of relevant bodies in Great Britain who can provide information about courses and local practitioners, and is correct as of Autumn 1989.

□ TENS

Make enquiries first to your local obstetric physiotherapist, who may already have suitable equipment and expertise. The major manufacturers, who advertise in midwifery or physiotherapy journals, will often provide research articles. They supply full instructions with their machines, and some run hire schemes for mothers.
   Half-day courses on diverse applications of TENS are held by:
The Centre For The Study Of Complementary Medicine
51 Bedford Place, Southampton, Hampshire SO1 2DG
Tel. (0703) 334752

□ Acupuncture

International College of Oriental Medicine, UK
Green Hedges House, Green Hedges Avenue, East Grinstead, East Sussex RH19 1DZ
Tel. (0342) 313106
This institution runs a three year full-time course for health practitioners, and publishes the International Register of Oriental Medicine

Traditional Acupuncture Society
1 The Ridgeway, Stratford-upon-Avon, Warwickshire CV37 9JL
Tel. (0789) 298798
Traditional Chinese approach. Runs comprehensive part-time courses for lay or paramedical personnel.

The British Acupuncture Association and Register
34 Alderney Street, London SW1V 4EU
Tel. 071-834 1012
Members are all qualified doctors or paramedics – for example nurses, physiotherapists, osteopaths.

The British Academy Of Western Acupuncture
Principal: Dr(Ac) R H Kay, Carrick, Tetchill, Ellesmere, Shropshire SY12 9AP
Tel (clinic). (0691) 654786
Organises six month courses for paramedics in pain relief techniques, mainly for musculo-skeletal disorders, and publishes a register of members.

☐ **Hypnosis**

The British Society Of Medical and Dental Hypnosis
Dr H Samuels (Honorary Secretary), 151 Otley Old Road, Leeds 16
The society holds a list of doctors and dentists practising hypnosis, which is available to health professionals.

British Society Of Experimental and Clinical Hypnosis
Department of Psychology, Middlewood Hospital, Sheffield S6 1TP
This organisation can provide names of local practitioners, also training for specific applications – for example, midwifery.

☐ **Homoeopathy**

Faculty of Homoeopathy, The Royal London Homoeopathic Hospital
Great Ormond Street, London WC1N 3HR
Tel. 071–837 8833
The faculty holds a register of over 700 medically trained homoeopaths. Educational activities include seminars for midwives.

☐ **Herbalism**

National Institute Of Medical Herbalists
Secretary: Janet Hicks, 41 Hatherly Rd, Winchester, Hants SO22 6RR
Tel. (0962) 68776
Can provide register and leaflets. The comprehensive course lasts four years, full-time or part-correspondence, for those with or without medical qualifications.

Bach Flower Remedies
Mount Vernon, Sotwell, Wallingford, Oxon OX10 0PZ

☐ **General**

Institute for Complementary Medicine
Interim address: 21 Portland Place, London W1N 3AS
Tel. 071–636 9543
A charity which carries updated details of all organisations relating to complementary medicine, and produces the British Register Of Alternative Practitioners. It plans to run courses for nurses on such subjects as massage and aromatherapy.

Chapter 6

Spontaneous delivery

Jennifer Sleep

Most mothers wish to achieve the safe and gentle delivery of their babies whilst retaining their own self esteem and the admiration and respect of their partners. This is especially true as delivery approaches when the pace of activity changes and excitement and anticipation mount. This is the time when a woman feels most vulnerable and dependent upon the influence of those privileged to share the experience. It is therefore the responsibility of professional attendants to safeguard her expectations of a spontaneous delivery by protecting the normal processes from unjustified intervention. In over 75 per cent of births in the UK this professional attendant will be the midwife (RCM 1987). It is she, therefore, who must accept this custodial role.

This chapter sets out to explore that role in the light of current research evidence by reviewing selected aspects of care during the second stage of labour. Some of this evidence has been generated by midwives themselves indicating their courage to question established practices and their commitment to improving the birth experience for the woman, her baby and her partner.

The issues to be discussed include the onset and duration of the second stage of labour, pushing policies, the choice of position for delivery, perineal management and perineal repair. Spontaneous delivery with minimal trauma will be considered the primary outcome of care.

■ It is assumed that you are already aware of the following:

- The physiological changes accompanying the second stage of labour;

- The anatomy of the pelvic floor;

- The action of anaesthetic drugs used for local infiltration.

■ The onset of the second stage

The second stage of labour begins when the cervix is fully dilated and ends with the birth of the baby. Functionally this stage may be reached without the mother's awareness, or may occur abruptly heralded by a dramatic change in the pace and intensity of contractions.

The woman may signal the transition to the second stage by a change in her breathing pattern or in the expression on her face or by increased restlessness. If the fetal head is visible at the introitus then full dilatation is easily confirmed. Up to two-thirds of women, however, feel the urge to bear down before this stage has been reached (Roberts *et al* 1987). In such an event, it is probably appropriate to check cervical dilatation by vaginal examination so that if 2–3 cms of cervix remains palpable, the woman may be encouraged to adopt a position in which she feels most comfortable and encouraged to resist this expulsive urge. If, however, only a rim of cervix is left and the woman is unable to resist her pushing urge, she may feel better by following her inclinations as long as she does not exhaust herself. There is little evidence that any harm will result (Roberts *et al* 1987).

■ Duration of the second stage

Documentation of the time of onset of the second stage is customary practice. This is often used as the basis for setting arbitrary time limits on its duration. A national survey in England found that limits of one hour for nulliparae and half an hour for multiparae were common policies (Garcia *et al* 1986). There is no good evidence, however, that when a labour is progressive and the condition of mother and fetus are satisfactory, that the imposition of an upper time limit improves outcome. The adverse sequelae attributed to prolonged second stage are consequent upon underlying causative factors, not on the absolute duration. Operative delivery may be required because of malpresentation, cephalo-pelvic disproportion, fetal or maternal distress but not simply because labour is prolonged. Indeed, if used inappropriately, assisting delivery may result in the very outcomes it is intended to prevent.

Only one trial has been published to date comparing two policies for curtailing the second stage in circumstances when the condition of mother and baby were satisfactory and the use of forceps or ventouse assistance was not elective. Twenty-two women whose babies' heads had become visible at the vulva were randomly allocated to either active encouragement to push and the liberal use of episiotomy or a more conservative approach (Wood *et al* 1973). Mean umbilical arterial pH values were statistically significantly higher in the 'active' group than the control group (7.28 as opposed to 7.23). It is important, however, to distinguish between statistical significance and clinical significance, as in this trial both values were within normal limits therefore posing no immediate threat to fetal wellbeing.

Retrospective studies do suggest, however, that limiting the duration of the second stage may modify the decline in the fetal pH which can occur over time (Roemer *et al* 1976). This may simply reflect a decrease in maternal pH levels during expulsion, without attendant risk to either fetus or mother. Without good evidence to suggest that limiting the duration of the second stage reduces obviously undesirable outcomes, such a policy cannot be justified (Alexander *et al* 1985). If the condition of both mother and baby are satisfactory and progress is occurring, there are no grounds for intervention.

■ Position for delivery

The position a mother may choose to adopt can be influenced by a combination of several factors including:

- Her personal preference;

- Her own and her baby's well-being;

- The place of delivery;

- The attitude and confidence of the attendant midwife.

In recent years both midwives and mothers have increasingly questioned the recumbent positions that women have been expected to adopt when giving birth in the hospital setting. Mothers have demanded greater flexibility in the attitude of professional carers and consideration of their personal choices. Many midwives have responded by developing their clinical skills and entering into a mutually consultative partnership with the women in their care.

Concerns about the problems related to the recumbent posture appear to be justified. The dorsal position carries a higher risk of supine hypotension due to aortocaval compression and a decrease in fetal oxygenation (Kurtz *et al* 1982). A 15° lateral tilt appears to reduce both these risks (Humphrey *et al* 1973).

The half sitting and supine positions during the second stage of labour were compared in a randomised trial of 100 women (Marttila *et al* 1983). Overall, the duration of labour was very similar in the two groups but there was a greater incidence of early decelerations in the fetal heart rate in the mothers who adopted the supine position. Ninety-eight per cent of the women in this study received elective episiotomies. Other studies suggest that a more upright posture can reduce the incidence of perineal trauma/episiotomy (Hillan 1983) and the need for assisted delivery (Liddell 1985). It should be noted, though, that the design and introduction of birthing chairs as a means of achieving this position has raised disquieting issues. In two randomised trials in which delivery in the birthing chair was compared with delivery in the conventional recumbent position, an increased risk of post-partum haemorrhage was reported in the groups using the birthing chair (Stewart *et al* 1983; Turner *et al* 1986). It seems unlikely that increased bleeding from the placental site is the causative factor; it is more likely to be consequent upon perineal trauma to tissues which have become engorged due to obstructed venous return. Observations of excessive perineal oedema and haemorrhoids in women who were upright in birthing chairs for extended periods of time help to substantiate this possible explanation (Cottrell & Shannahan 1986).

In some of these studies, mothers have been asked their views on these various positions. Overall they responded more positively to the upright posture, reporting less pain (Marttila *et al* 1983), and a desire to use a similar position in subsequent labours (Hemminki *et al* 1986). The midwives' opinions were also considered in two trials. In the study conducted by Stewart *et al* (1983), the use of the chair was reported to be 'satisfactory' whilst Hemminki and colleagues (1986) suggested that the midwives' assessment depended strongly upon their initial attitude towards the chair which remained unchanged upon completion of the study. They therefore concluded that the skill and confidence of the midwife may be more important than the chair itself.

The squatting position also has its advocates. Russell (1982) used radiological evidence to review the anatomical forces acting on the pelvis when the trunk is vertical and the thighs abducted. The pelvic outlet was increased by as much as 28 per cent offering considerable potential advantages to the ease of delivery. Such observations lend support to the anthropological evidence that the squatting posture may be favourable for delivery. However, no formal evaluation of this position has yet been conducted.

Overall, the current evidence suggests that women may be encouraged to adopt a whole range of differing positions for delivery without compromising their babies' health or their own wellbeing. It is interesting to note that in Garcia's (1986) survey, although 87 per cent of consultant units reported that women were able to choose their delivery position, 74 per cent of the women opted for the semi-recumbent posture. This may reflect 'Hobson's choice', for unless women are offered a preparatory exercise and education programme during pregnancy, endorsed by positive encouragement to experiment with alternative positions during labour they are unlikely to feel sufficiently confident to follow their own inclinations.

■ Pushing

One of the major considerations in the conduct of the second stage, is whether the time honoured practice of actively encouraging maternal pushing successfully speeds the time to delivery with any good effect. Most women eventually experience an overwhelming urge to push at some time during the expulsive phase of labour. When this occurs little can, or should, effectively be done to control her involuntary efforts. What is in question is whether she needs, or should be given, formal instruction to practice sustained breath holding during directed, strenuous pushing effort; that is to practice the Valsalva manoeuvre. In a small study comparing this manoeuvre with the use of the exhalation-pushing technique, the incidence of fetal heart rate abnormality was greater when the women practised sustained breath holding; the mean duration of the second stage was similar in the two groups (Knauth & Haloburdo 1986).

In an observational study Caldeyro-Barcia (1979) described directed pushing efforts which lasted approximately three times longer than self regulated pushing; potentially harmful haemodynamic consequences may result particularly when the woman is in the supine position. These adverse consequences include aorto-caval compression and reduced blood flow to the uterus and lower limbs (Bassell *et al* 1980).

When epidural anaesthesia has been administered maternal bearing down efforts are modified either by the anaesthetic (which tends to reduce or delay them), or by the caregivers (who tend to encourage them). The effect of encouraging earlier pushing in these circumstances has been evaluated in two randomised trials (McQueen & Mylrea 1977; Maresh *et al* 1983). In both of these studies rotational forceps deliveries were more common amongst those women who had been encouraged to bear down relatively early and in neither study was there any evidence that this policy had any compensating advantages for either the mother or the baby.

Despite the limitations of the available evidence, a fairly consistent pattern emerges. Although the widespread policy of directing women to use sustained and early pushing effort may well result in a modest decrease in the duration of the second stage, these policies may compromise maternal-fetal gas exchange, increase the risk of instrumental delivery and consequently, as Benyon (1957) suggested, perineal damage.

■ Prevention of perineal trauma

As the moment of birth approaches and the fetal head begins to distend the perineum, policies of care are directed towards the best method of preventing and minimising soft tissue trauma. Several antecedent factors can influence perineal outcome, namely the quantity and timing of analgesia/anaesthesia, the total duration of labour and the condition of both mother and fetus. This is, however, the time when midwifery skills, enhanced by mutual trust and respect between midwife and mother, can play an important role in securing a gentle, controlled and safe delivery with minimal trauma to the woman or her baby. Preventing perineal trauma is particularly important because it can cause pain and discomfort which may dominate the experience of early motherhood and have far reaching consequences for both the woman and her partner (Kitzinger 1981).

Physical methods designed to prevent trauma are based on the belief that the tissues may be stretched and rendered more supple either by the use of massage during the prenatal or immediate pre-delivery period or by the process of 'ironing out' the perineum as the second stage advances. Warm compresses or emollients such as olive oil, walnut or almond oils may be used, as well as herbal preparations for example, calendula cream containing extract of marigold. These therapies may be carried out by the woman, her partner or the attendant midwife. Such practices have enthusiastic advocates (Flint 1986); others are more sceptical suggesting that touch may prove a distraction, creating tension as well as increasing vascularity and oedema in tissues already at risk from trauma (Noble 1983). Neither of these polarised opinions can be supported by research evidence. Only two published studies have attempted to evaluate the use of perineal massage (Avery & Burket 1986; Avery & Van Arsdale 1987). Unfortunately, the methodological weaknesses and small sample size in each of the trials (in the first the number was 20, in the second 55) does not offer results which can be helpful in guiding midwifery practice. The use of oral herbal remedies such as arnica tablets (to reduce bruising) also remains unevaluated.

Guarding the perineum is a time honoured practice where the attendant's hand held against the perineum during contractions is believed to support the tissues, thus minimising the risk of spontaneous trauma. In reality, it is difficult to see how exerting such limited external pressure can circumvent the enormous internal pressure which accompanies expulsive contractions. The prophylactic principle is more logical when applied to the practice of exerting gentle pressure to the fetal head as a means of controlling the speed of 'crowning' as this is when the perineal tissues are most at risk of spontaneous damage.

☐ The use of episiotomy

The most common cause of perineal damage is episiotomy. A review of the English language literature from 1860 to 1980 (Thacker & Banta 1983) stated that this procedure is carried out on between 50 and 90 per cent of women giving birth to their first child. The authors further suggested that the three postulated benefits of a liberal episiotomy policy had not been adequately substantiated by available research evidence. These benefits include prevention of damage to the anal sphincter, prevention of trauma to the fetal head and prevention of serious damage to the muscles of the pelvic floor. As a surgical operation the procedure carries a number of risks including haemorrhage and infection as well as the attendant risk of extension of the incision to involve the anal sphincter and rectal mucosa – injuries which are less likely to occur as a consequence of spontaneous trauma (Thorp *et al* 1987).

There would seem to be little controversy relating to the use of episiotomy for fetal indications, but the rationale for its routine use for maternal reasons in otherwise normal deliveries is disputed. The differing policies of perineal management based on maternal indications have been compared in two experimental studies. Harrison and colleagues (1984) randomly allocated 181 primiparae to one of two policies on admission in labour. The liberal episiotomy group received elective intervention. Women allocated to the restricted policy were allowed to deliver without intervention unless severe spontaneous trauma or fetal problems were anticipated. The resultant episiotomy rate was 8 per cent. The subsequent analyses were based on only 77 women and so are subject to selection bias. Perineal pain was assessed during the first four days after delivery and at six weeks post partum. In the second study, Sleep and her colleagues (1984) compared two policies for perineal management aimed to minimise trauma during spontaneous vaginal deliveries; both primiparae and multiparae were recruited to the study. Five hundred and two women were randomly allocated to the liberal episiotomy policy (the procedure being used selectively either to prevent a tear or when there was evidence of fetal compromise); 498 women were allocated to the restricted policy (intended to limit episiotomy to fetal indications only). The resultant episiotomy rates were 51 per cent and 10 per cent respectively. All analyses were based on all the women allocated to the two policies regardless of subsequent management as this is free from selection bias.

There was no significant difference in neonatal outcome based on Apgar score at delivery and the number of babies needing admission to SCBU.

At the time of delivery, the liberal use of episiotomy was associated with more perineal trauma overall and there was no evidence that this policy substantially reduced the risk of serious trauma to either the upper vagina or to the anal sphincter and rectal mucosa. There was some suggestion that it was protective against anterior labial tears. At both 10 days and at three months post partum the two groups reported a comparable amount of perineal pain. Although women allocated to the liberal policy resumed intercourse somewhat later than those in the restricted group, the proportions of women experiencing painful intercourse three months and three years after delivery was almost identical (Sleep & Grant 1987).

The hypothesis that liberal use of episiotomy protects against the subsequent development of urinary incontinence has been tested in a longer term follow up (Sleep & Grant 1987). In the three month assessment described in the original paper, overall 19 per cent of women reported some measure of urinary incontinence. Three years later the overall prevalence had increased to 35 per cent but there was little difference in the rate and severity of incontinence in the women originally allocated to the two trial groups.

Neither of these trials provides evidence that conducting episiotomies liberally in order to prevent tears will offer women any benefits. The routine use of episiotomy is therefore not justified.

☐ Midline versus medio-lateral episiotomy

In both of the above trials, the medio-lateral incision was used. This is the most popular form of operation in the UK, as it is believed to reduce the risks of extension of the incision into the anal sphincter (Pritchard & MacDonald 1980). The midline incision is far more common in North America. Its claimed advantages include lower risk of third degree extension, reduced blood loss, ease of repair, better healing and less post partum pain and dyspareunia (Pritchard & MacDonald 1980). These two approaches have been compared in only one randomised trial (Coats *et al* 1980). Third degree lacerations occurred in 39 of 163 women (24 per cent) in the midline episiotomy group and in only 22 of 193 (9 per cent) in those who received a medio-lateral incision. The perineum was significantly less bruised in the women who had had the midline operation but the amount of pain experienced was similar in the two groups, as were the proportions of women requiring analgesia. Women in the midline episiotomy group began intercourse significantly earlier than those who had medio-lateral incisions. At follow up the investigators judged the cosmetic appearance and texture of the scar to be somewhat better following the midline operation. The womens' opinion was not sought, however, so important, long term outcome measures such as the incidence of dyspareunia, urinary or faecal incontinence were not addressed. This small study provides the only evidence to date to evaluate two differing approaches to a practice which can have major implications for the lives of women and their partners.

☐ Local anaesthetics for perineal infiltration

A prerequisite to perineal repair is the provision of an adequate level of anaesthesia for the mother. There is, however, little available evidence to support a particular choice of anaesthetic for perineal infiltration. The general principle is to give the smallest effective dose in the lowest concentration. Lignocaine hydrochloride (Xylocaine) and prilocaine (Citanest), both in a one per cent solution, appear to be most commonly used in maternity units. Each agent has a relatively rapid onset of action (approximately 3–4 minutes), the anaesthetic effect lasting approximately for one hour. There appears to be little consensus of opinion whether or not they should be used in combination with adrenaline.

The addition of adrenaline causes vasoconstriction which offers an advantage in a highly vascular area such as the perineum where the solution might otherwise be quickly carried away from the site of injection. The absorption and anaesthetic effect are not delayed but the overall duration of action is extended. The disadvantage of adrenaline lies in its toxicity if accidentally administered intravenously; these effects include tinnitus, confusion and light headedness (Moore 1983).

Bupivacaine (Marcain) offers the advantage of long action, (approximately 3–4 hours) but delayed onset (10–30 minutes); it is therefore not the anaesthetic of choice and cannot be combined with Lignocaine to provide the best of both worlds – that is to say a quick acting, long duration anaesthetic (Martindale 1989). The dearth of research evidence to assess the effectiveness of agents offers considerable scope for further studies.

If an effective epidural is in progress, this may ensure that the woman is pain free; one recent trial however, suggests that such mothers may also benefit from local infiltration as a means of distending the tissues prior to suturing (Khan & Lilford 1987). In this study, pain in the first 24 hours was significantly reduced and analgesic requirements were less for mothers who received infiltration prior to repair.

☐ **Perineal repair**

Over 69 per cent of mothers sustain perineal trauma requiring repair by suturing following spontaneous delivery which means that every day in England and Wales about 1000 women are likely to need perineal repair after childbirth (Sleep *et al* 1984). The majority of these will be sutured by midwives (Garcia *et al* 1986). There are three main considerations; the choice of suture material, the technique of repair and the competence of the operator. A recent survey of 50 maternity units revealed 13 different combinations of suture materials used for the deeper tissues and the skin; when absorbable materials were chosen half the units used interrupted technique, 7 per cent used continuous subcuticular suturing, the remainder using the two techniques equally (Grant 1986). This evidence demonstrates the lack of current consensus as to the best choice of materials and suturing technique for skin closure.

Fourteen controlled trials have been published to date; these have been well reviewed by Grant (1989). Basically, the choice of suture material rests between threads which absorb over a period of time or those which require removal in the early postnatal period. The advantage of absorbable material is that the same thread can be used to repair all the tissue layers. Two absorbable materials have been compared in a number of studies, namely polyglycolic acid (marketed as Dexon and as Vicryl) and chromic catgut. Overall, polyglycolic acid was associated with about 40 per cent reduction in pain and the need for analgesia in the short term. The main criticism of this material, however, was that the thread often needs removal as long as three months following delivery (Mahomed *et al* 1989). This is the only reported study in which a longer term follow up of women has been successfully conducted. Polyglycolic acid sutures seemed to reduce the need for re-suturing but also to be associated with a later resumption of intercourse. Of the women who had resumed intercourse at three months post partum, the incidence of dyspareunia was no greater than those sutured using other materials.

One study (Spencer *et al* 1986) which did include both short and longer term follow up compared glycerol-impregnated catgut (Braun Softgut) with chromic catgut for all the layers. Pain on the tenth day was 37 per cent more common and dyspareunia in the first three months after delivery was 26 per cent more common in the women repaired with softgut, than in the group repaired using chromic catgut. This difference persisted three years later when intercourse was 1.7 times more often reported as painful by women repaired with softgut (Grant 1989). Extrapolation of these results to England and Wales would suggest that the choice of suture material could make a difference of as many as 30 000 cases of dyspareunia each year (Grant 1986).

Nonabsorbable skin sutures (silk and nylon) have been compared with absorbable materials (catgut and polyglycolic acid) in only six studies (Hansen *et al* 1975; Gaasemyr *et al* 1977; Brendsel & Madsen 1980; Buchan & Nicholls 1980; Isager-Sally *et al* 1986; Mahomed *et al* 1989). In general, the groups repaired with polyglycolic acid sutures left to dissolve had less pain and used less analgesia in the first five days after delivery. There was no clear difference, however, in longer term pain or dyspareunia.

The choice of technique used in skin closure is also an important issue. Overall, the evidence to date suggests that interrupted sutures cause more pain both in the short and in the longer term than continuous subcuticular stitch to the skin (Isager-Sally 1986). Grant (1986) suggests, however, that this approach may be more suitable for the experienced operator, whilst the interrupted technique may cause fewer problems in the hands of the inexperienced or novice operator or for jagged tears.

Given this evidence it would seem that polyglycolic acid remains the material of choice for repair of all the tissue layers. Compared with catgut its use is associated with about a 40 per cent reduction in short term pain and the need for analgesia. Continuous subcuticular technique appears preferable to interrupted transcutaneous suturing, particularly in terms of perineal pain in the early puerperium (Grant 1989).

■ Recommendations for clinical practice in the light of currently available evidence

1. There is no good evidence to support the imposition of any arbitary time limit when the second stage of labour is progressing and the

condition of both mother and fetus is satisfactory. Such limits should therefore be discarded.

2. There are no data to suggest that women need to be taught how and when to push during the active stage. Indeed the practice of sustained breath holding and exerted pushing effort currently taught in many antenatal classes may be positively harmful to both the mother and her baby. Women should therefore be encouraged to follow their own inclinations to push as and when they feel the urge to do so.

3. The recumbent posture tends to lengthen the second stage of labour, to increase the incidence of abnormal fetal heart rate patterns and overall to reduce the number of spontaneous deliveries. Confining women to bed or restricting them to the use of the supine position for delivery is therefore unjustified.

4. The enthusiastic use of birthing chairs as a means of achieving an upright posture appears to predispose to perineal oedema, venous engorgement and increased risk of excessive blood loss. This is not the only way a mother may be supported in a more upright position, however. The use of wedges, bean bags, birthing bars, and the adoption of a variety of postures should be explored and assessed.

5. Prophylactic measures designed to reduce perineal trauma have been poorly evaluated. There is no evidence to support the use of herbal remedies or massage in maintaining perineal integrity, on the other hand none of these methods has been shown to be harmful. Their possible contribution to improving the outcome of labour merits more careful consideration and evaluation.

6. There is no evidence to support a policy of liberally using episiotomy as a means of reducing tears; the procedure should therefore be restricted to fetal indications only. The benefits and disadvantages of medio-lateral versus midline incision should be explored and also the use of scissors or scalpel for making the incision.

7. The action of various anaesthetic agents for local infiltration should be explored both with and without the addition of adrenaline.

8. Interrupted sutures as a method of skin closure in perineal repair may cause considerably more discomfort for women both in the short and longer term. Midwives who are initially taught this technique should progress to seek instruction and gain expertise in subcuticular technique. In addition, several of the suture materials recently marketed seem to be a major contributary factor in increasing pain and dyspareunia in women following childbirth. New products should not be introduced into clinical care without careful and thorough evaluation generated from the conduct of randomised controlled trials.

9. Overall, midwives need to gain confidence in their own ability to care for women throughout the course of normal labour and delivery with the minimum of intervention. Intelligent passivity is an art; to perfect it in practice requires clinical judgement based on perceptive observation and sound evidence, coupled with sensitivity and respect for individual preferences. Initially, this is not easy to achieve, but as professional confidence grows a unique mother/midwife partnership is forged. This relationship built on trust and skill culminates in a birth experience which is both joyful and fulfilling.

■ Practice check

- Does your unit currently have a policy stating an upper limit of duration of the second stage of labour? If so, when was this last reviewed or discussed by the midwives?

- Are women taught pushing techniques in antenatal classes in your district? Do the midwives who regularly conduct deliveries take part in these sessions? Do the women receive detailed information about perineal management during delivery – the alternative approaches and methods of repair currently practiced by you and your colleagues?

- How many episiotomies do you personally conduct per 100 deliveries? Are the indications documented in the mother's notes together with details of the technique and suture material used in the repair? Following a delivery, do you visit a mother on the postnatal ward to check that all is well?

- Who is responsible for teaching midwives to suture the perineum in your unit? Are there opportunities for updating skills or learning new techniques? Are midwives involved in discussions with obstetric colleagues with regard to choice of suturing threads?

□ Acknowledgements

The author gratefully acknowledges the support of colleagues at the National Perinatal Epidemiology Unit Oxford, in particular Dr Adrian Grant, Epidemiologist and Dr Iain Chalmers, Director.

■ References

Alexander S, Cantraine F, Schwers J 1985 Apgar score and cord pH in relation to length of second stage. In Rolfe P (ed) Fetal and neonatal physiological measurements: 59–64. Butterworths, London

Avery M D, Burket B A 1986 Effect of perineal massage on the incidence of episiotomy and perineal laceration in a nurse midwifery service. Journal of Nurse-Midwifery 31: 128–34

Avery M D, Van Arsdale L 1987 Perineal massage: effect on the incidence of episiotomy and laceration in a nulliparous population. Journal of Nurse-Midwifery 32(3): 181–84

Bassell G M, Humayun S G, Marx G F 1980 Maternal bearing down efforts – another fetal risk? Obstetrics and Gynecology 56: 39–41

Brendsel J, Madsen H 1980 Intracutaneous suturing of episiotomy wounds. Ugeskr Laeger 142: 3120–22

Buchan P C, Nicholls J A J 1980 Pain after episiotomy – a comparison of two methods of repair. Journal of the Royal College of General Practitioners 30: 297–300

Benyon C L 1957 The normal second stage of labour: a plea for reform in its conduct. Journal of Obstetrics and Gynaecology of the British Empire 64: 815–20

Caldeyro-Barcia R 1979 The influence of maternal bearing down efforts during second stage on fetal well being. Birth and the Family Journal 6(1): 17–21

Coats P M, Chan K K, Wilkins M, Beard R J 1980 A comparison between midline and mediolateral episiotomies. British Journal of Obstetrics and Gynaecology 87: 408–12

Cottrell B H, Shannahan M D 1986 Effect of the birth chair on duration of second stage labour and maternal outcome. Nursing Research 35: 364–67

Flint C 1986 Sensitive Midwifery. Heinemann, London: 101–02

Garcia J, Garforth S, Ayers S 1986 Midwives confined? Labour ward policies and routines: 74–80. Research and the Midwife Conference Proceedings, University of Manchester

Gaasemyr M, Hovland E, Bergsjo P 1977 Suturaterialets betydning for tilheling etter episiotomi – sammenlikning mellom cromcatgut og supramid. Fra Medisinske Publikasjoner 2: 1–5

Grant A 1986 Repair of episiotomies and perineal tears. British Journal of Obstetrics and Gynaecology 93: 417–19

Grant A 1989 The choice of suture materials and techniques for repair of perineal trauma: an overview of the evidence from controlled trials. British Journal of Obstetrics and Gynaecology 96(11): 1281–89

Hansen M K, Selnes A, Simonsen E, Sorensen K M, Pederson G T 1975 Polyglycolic acid (Dexon) used as suture material for the repair of episiotomies. Ugeskr Laeger 137: 617–20

Harrison R F, Brennan M, North P M, Reed J V, Wickham E A 1984 Is routine episiotomy necessary? British Medical Journal 288: 1971–75

Hillan E 1983 The birthing chair trial. Research and the Midwife Conference Proceedings, University of Manchester

Hemminki E, Virkkunen A, Makela A, Hannikainen J, Pulkkis E, Moilanen K, Pasanen M 1986 A trial of delivery in a birth chair. Journal of Obstetrics and Gynaecology 6: 162–5

Humphrey M, Hounslow D, Morgan S, Wood C 1973 The influence of maternal posture at birth on the fetus. Journal of Obstetrics and Gynaecology British Commonwealth 80: 1075–80

Kitzinger S 1981 Some women's experiences of episiotomies. National Childbirth Trust, London

Knauth D G, Haloburdo E P 1986 Effect of pushing techniques in birthing chair on length of second stage labour. Nursing Research 35: 49–51

Kurz C S, Schneider H, Huch R, Huch A 1982 The influence of the maternal position on the fetal transcutaneous oxygen pressure (tcpO$_2$). Journal of Perinatal Medicine 10 (Supplement 2): 74–5

Isager-Sally L, Legarth J, Jacobson B, Bustofte E 1986 Episiotomy repair – immediate and long term sequelae. A prospective randomised study of three different methods of repair. British Journal of Obstetrics and Gynaecology 93: 420–25

Khan G, Lilford R J 1987 Wound pain may be reduced by prior infiltration of the episiotomy, site after delivery under epidural anaesthesia. British Journal of obstetrics and Gynaecologists 94: 341–44

Liddell H S, Fisher P R 1985 The birthing chair in the second stage of labour. Australian and New Zealand Journal of Obstetrics and Gynaecology 25: 65–8

Mahomed K, Grant A, Ashburst H, James D 1989 The Southmead perineal suture study. British Journal of Obstetrics and Gynaecology 96(11): 1272–80

Maresh M, Choong K H, Beard R W 1983 Delayed pushing with lumbar epidural analgesia in labour. British Journal of Obstetrics and Gynaecology 90: 623–27

Martindale 1989 Extra pharmacopoeia: 1205–27. Pharmaceutical Press, London

Marttila M, Kajanoja P, Ylikorkala O 1983 Maternal half sitting position in the second stage of labour. Journal of Perinatal Medicine 11: 286–91

McQueen J, Mylrea L 1977 Lumbar epidural analgesia in labour. British Medical Journal 1: 640–41

Moore D C 1983 Systemic toxicity of local anaesthetic drugs. Seminars in Anaesthesia (Regional Anesthesia) 2: 62–74

Noble E 1983 Childbirth with insight: 88. Houghton Mifflin, Boston

Pritchard J A, MacDonald P C (eds) 1980 Williams Obstetrics, 16th ed. Appleton Century Crofts, New York

Roberts J E, Goldstein S A, Gruener J S, Maggio M, Mendez-Bauer C 1987 A descriptive analysis of involuntary bearing down efforts during the expulsive phase of labour. Journal of Obstetrics, Gynecology and Neonatal Nursing 16: 48–55

Roemer V M, Harms K, Buess H, Horvath T J 1976 Response of fetal acid-base balance to duration of second stage of labour. International Journal of Obstetrics and Gynaecology 14: 455–71

Royal College of Midwives 1987 Towards a healthy nation. RCM policy document for the maternity services. RCM, London

Russell J G 1982 The rationale of primitive delivery positions. British Journal of Obstetrics and Gynaecology 89: 712–15

Sleep J M, Grant A, Garcia J, Elbourne D, Spencer J, Chalmers I 1984 West Berkshire perineal management trial. British Medical Journal 289: 587–90

Sleep J, Grant A 1987 West Berkshire perineal management trial: three year follow up. British Medical Journal 295: 749–51

Spencer J A D, Grant A, Elbourne D, Garcia J, Sleep J 1986 A randomised comparison of glycerol impregnated chromic catgut with untreated chromic catgut for the repair of perineal trauma. British Journal of Obstetrics and Gynaecology 93: 426–30

Stewart P, Hillan E, Calder A A 1983 A randomised trial to evaluate the use of a birth chair for delivery. Lancet i: 1296–8

Thacker S E, Banta H D 1983 Benefits and risks of episiotomy: and interpretative review of the English language literature, 1860–1980. Obstetrical and Gynaecological Survey 38: 322–38

Thorp J M, Bowes W A, Brame R G, Cefalo R 1987 Selected use of midline episiotomy: effect on perineal trauma. Obstetrics and Gynecology 70: 260–2

Turner M J, Romney M L, Webb J B, Gordon H 1986 The birthing chair: an obstetric hazard? Journal of Obstetrics and Gynaecology 6: 232–35

Wood C, Ng K H, Hounslow D, Benning H 1973 Time – an important variable in normal delivery. Journal of Obstetrics and Gynaecology of the British Commonwealth 80: 295–300

■ Suggested further reading

Gardosi J, Sylvester S, Lynch C B 1989 Alternative positions in the second stage of labour: a randomised controlled trial. British Journal of Obstetrics and Gynaecology 96(11): 1290–96

Grant A 1989 Repair of perineal trauma after childbirth. In Chalmers I, Erkin M, Kierse M (eds) Effective care in pregnancy and childbirth: 1129–44. Oxford University Press, Oxford

Sleep J. Roberts J, Chalmers I 1989 Care during the Second stage of labour. In Chalmers I, Enkin M, Kierse M (eds) Effective care in pregnancy and childbirth: 1129–44. Oxford University Press, Oxford

Chapter 7

The midwife's management of the third stage of labour

Valerie Levy

This chapter concerns the midwife's management of the third stage of labour. Optimum management of the third stage implies the following.

1. Antenatal care that enables the mother to enter the third stage of labour in:
   – the appropriate place (for example, a consultant unit if she is 'at risk');
   – as healthy a condition as possible (for example, with an adequate haemoglobin level in order to withstand blood loss).

2. Good management of the first and second stages of labour so that the mother enters the third stage with a uterus capable of contracting and retracting.

3. Good management of the third stage of labour so that the placenta and membranes are delivered complete and haemorrhage is minimal. During this time the umbilical cord is clamped and cut, and the relationship between the baby and the mother and probably the father will start, or continue.

Postpartum haemorrhage is recognised as the most common serious complication of the third stage. Although it is difficult to obtain accurate local and national statistics, commonly quoted postpartum haemorrhage rates following normal deliveries vary between 5 and 7 per cent.

The consequences of postpartum haemorrhage are sometimes minimal, but occasionally devastating. In the triennium 1982 to 1984, three women in England and Wales died as a direct result of postpartum haemorrhage (DHSS 1989). This was the lowest figure recorded in any triennium, but it was noted that haemorrhage had contributed to other deaths which were directly attributed to other causes.

The management of the third stage tends to focus upon the prevention of postpartum haemorrhage, and much of this chapter concentrates upon this aspect.

Policies of 'active' management have been formulated to prevent haemorrhage, but the efficacy of these policies has recently been challenged and re-examined. This chapter will present some of the arguments and research directed towards assessing the value of active management, and will suggest additions to the lists of risk factors for postpartum haemorrhage traditionally quoted in textbooks.

Factors relating to mother-baby interaction during the third stage will not be discussed in this chapter, which will concentrate almost exclusively upon the purely maternal aspects of the third stage. The management of abnormalities such as haemorrhage will not be included, nor will issues outside the midwife's usual sphere of practice.

■ It is assumed that you are already aware of the following:

- The anatomy of the placenta and membranes;

- The physiology of placental separation;

- The principles of active and 'physiological' management of the third stage of labour;

- The possible complications of the third stage, and their management;

- The mechanisms of neonatal jaundice.

■ The management of the third stage of labour

Cord traction is by no means a recent innovation in the management of the third stage of labour; 2000 years ago Aristotle advocated cord traction to 'bring away the after-burden, for it can prove dangerous if it be not speedily done' (Hibbard 1964). In more recent years cord traction was used less as the principles of cross infection became understood. Other methods were used instead, none of which necessitated handling the cord close to the genitalia, such as Crede's manoeuvre, fundal pressure, or of course, delivery by maternal effort. Some of these methods undoubtedly prolonged the duration of the third stage, but length was not an unduly critical factor until the introduction of prophylactic oxytocics.

□ Oxytocics

In the 1930s, ergometrine was identified as the active oxytocic component of ergot and its use for the prevention and control of postpartum haemorrhage became widespread. Synthetic oxytocin was developed in the 1950s, and Embrey *et al* (1963) recommended the use of a combined preparation of ergometrine and syntocinon (Syntometrine) in order to combine the benefits of the slower acting but sustained action of ergometrine, and the quicker, shorter lasting action of syntocinon; Syntometrine began to be widely used in Britain during the 1960s.

Oxytocics are now commonly used in the management of the third stage, but although their value in the control of postpartum haemorrhage is acknowledged they are not without side-effects including hypertension, headache, nausea and vomiting. Their routine prophylactic use has consequently been challenged by consumer groups, midwives and other professionals.

In order to assess the value of prophylactic oxytocics, Prendiville *et al* (1988a) reviewed nine published controlled trials. The combined data from these studies indicated that the prophylactic use of oxytocics reduces the risk of postpartum haemorrhage by 40 per cent and the rate of postpartum haemorrhage from 10 per cent to 6 per cent. As Prendiville acknowledges however, these nine trials provide imprecise descriptions of the management of the third stage and the data is consequently of limited value. Further controlled trials are needed, but in the interim the indications are that the prophylactic use of oxytocics reduces postpartum haemorrhage.

Elbourne *et al* (1988) reviewed data from 27 controlled trials to assess the relative benefits of ergot preparations, oxytocin, prostaglandins and Syntometrine. They concluded that there is little justification for the sole use of ergot preparations (such as ergonovine or ergometrine) in the management of the third stage; not only are they no more effective than other oxytocics, but there are greater side effects particularly regarding hypertension. Indeed, Prendiville *et al* (1988a) recommend that the use of oxytocics should be considered carefully in cardiovascularly compromised women. There was insufficient data to compare the incidences of nausea, vomiting and headache.

Elbourne and her colleagues found Syntometrine to be more effective in reducing postpartum haemorrhage than oxytocin alone (albeit at a greater risk of hypertension). They emphasised the need for a large controlled trial however, in order to properly compare Syntometrine with oxytocin in terms of reducing blood loss, and to more accurately assess their relative effects on hypertension and unpleasant symptoms such as vomiting.

☐ **Controlled cord traction**

Ergometrine causes spasm of the lower segment and cervix (Sorbe 1978), which can result in entrapment of the placenta and the consequent associated complications of postpartum haemorrhage and manual removal. The administration of ergometrine (or Syntometrine) therefore necessitates prompt delivery of the placenta by cord traction and this is the method of placental delivery now most commonly used in Britain and many other developed countries.

'Controlled' cord traction seems to have first been described by Spencer (1962). Spencer expressed her concern about high postpartum haemorrhage rates and subsequently conducted a trial of controlled cord traction in 1000 mothers, delivered normally. (The exact method of third stage management employed prior to this study is not clear.)

Mothers participating in the trial were given intravenous ergometrine (500 micrograms) at the birth of the anterior shoulder, the baby was delivered slowly and the cord divided. When the uterus was well contracted, the left hand of the accoucher was placed on the lower abdomen and the lower segment grasped between the index finger and thumb, and steady pressure exerted in a backwards and upwards direction in order to exactly counterbalance the simultaneous traction applied to the cord, so that the position of the uterus in the abdomen remained unchanged. Traction on the cord was gentle at first, but gradually increased until delivery of the placenta was achieved; if controlled cord traction was unsuccessful at first the procedure was repeated every few minutes.

Spencer emphasised that the 'classical' signs of placental separation were *not* to be awaited, but controlled cord traction was to be applied as soon as the uterus was contracted. This she considered to be quite safe as long as the uterus was indeed contracted and it was supported in position in the abdomen by the accoucheur's left hand.

By implementing this technique, Spencer found the mean blood loss to be 90 ml and the mean length of the third stage just over six minutes. The postpartum haemorrhage rate was approximately one per cent and the manual removal rate two per cent (half the women experiencing postpartum haemorrhage required manual removal, a result which she considered disappointing).

This was not a controlled trial however and comparisons are impossible between controlled cord traction and other methods of third stage management. This uncontrolled trial was apparently greatly influential in changing the management of the third stage of labour (certainly in Great Britain, and very probably elsewhere).

There followed a long absence of published work to assess the effects of controlled cord traction; the medical and midwifery literature between 1961 and the early 1980s is almost silent on the relative merits of controlled cord traction, fundal pressure and maternal effort in the management of the third stage of labour. Most relevant research during this time is concerned with the benefits of various oxytocics.

☐ **'Active' versus 'physiological' management**

The purpose of active management is to shorten the third stage, thus reducing the risk of haemorrhage; also, less midwifery time is required. The benefits of active management have recently been questioned however, notably by Inch (1983; 1985) who describes the resultant 'cascade of intervention' when the normal physiological processes of placental separation and descent are hastened.

A randomised controlled trial has recently compared the outcomes of active and physiological third stage management (Prendiville *et al* 1988b). The trial took place in a major obstetric unit where active management was the policy. Eight hundred and forty-six women were randomly allocated to the 'active' management group; active management involved the administration of an oxytocic with the birth of the anterior shoulder, clamping the cord 30 seconds after delivery, and applying controlled cord traction when the uterus had contracted. Eight hundred and forty-nine women were allocated to the 'physiological' group; no oxytocic was given, controlled cord traction was *not* used and the fundus not manipulated. The mother was encouraged to adopt an upright position to aid delivery of the placenta by gravity; maternal effort only was used. If the placenta was not delivered spontaneously then the baby was put to the breast and maternal effort further encouraged. If problems arose, this protocol was adapted to individual circumstances.

In the 'physiological' group, the cord was left unclamped and attached to the baby until the placenta was delivered. Inch (1983; 1985) suggests that if the cord is clamped immediately after delivery then blood, which would otherwise have been drained away, remains in the placenta and renders it incapable of becoming compact and compressed. Retraction is thereby prevented, placental separation slowed, and blood loss increased.

In the group of mothers whose third stages were managed actively, their third stages were shorter (median length five minutes in the active group compared to 15 minutes in the physiological group), the postpartum haemorrhage rate was less (5.9 per cent as opposed to 17.9 per cent), there were fewer blood transfusions and less need for therapeutic oxytocics. The results related to blood loss were supported by objective measurements of maternal haematocrits and haemoglobins.

The results were unaffected by whether the labour had been induced or augmented, or by the use of epidural blocks or instrumental delivery. Indeed, the trends were even more marked in the women who had had low risk, normal labours and deliveries.

Twice as many women in the active management group vomited (and there was an increase in the incidence of headaches and hypertension, although these differences were not statistically significant).

There were no statistically significant differences between the groups regarding manual removal of placenta, subsequent evacuation of retained products, or the length of stay in hospital. Nor were there statistically significant differences regarding neonatal Apgar scores or respiratory problems. Babies of mothers in the physiological group had a significantly higher haematocrit, and (although not statistically significant) a higher incidence of jaundice, and were more likely to require admission to the special care nursery.

The Unit's policy of active management was thereby considered justified. However, as the authors of this paper themselves point out, few of the midwives participating in this study were experienced in carrying out physiological management of the third stage and were given only a short time (six weeks) in which to become proficient in this 'new' type of management. The results may therefore have reflected the midwives' comparative lack of experience in physiological third stage management rather than problems inherent in the method itself. Furthermore, Harding (1988) comments that the midwives undertaking the deliveries may have been prejudiced against physiological third stages as these deliveries took longer and if they occurred at the end of a shift would have delayed the midwife. No overtime payment was available. Prendiville *et al* (1988b) suggest that the trial should be replicated 'in a setting in which physiological management is the norm'.

Physiological third stages are commonly practised at Hinchingbrooke Hospital. From 1986 to 1988, 15.4 per cent (906 out of 5861) women had physiological third stages. The postpartum haemorrhage rate in the physiological group was 7 per cent, compared to an overall postpartum haemorrhage rate of 7.6 per cent (Milner 1989).

Milner stresses that midwives who conduct physiological third stages must feel competent to do so, and no midwife at Hinchingbrooke is required to deliver a placenta in this way until she feels completely confident. Milner also points out that physiological delivery of the placenta should only be undertaken when the first and second stages have been completely normal – 'a natural delivery of the placenta is the logical culmination of a natural labour'.

Many midwives have comparatively little experience of alternative methods of delivering the placenta, particularly if they work in obstetric units where the policy is that of active management of the third stage. It is now common practice for Syntometrine to be administered prophylactically, together with controlled cord traction (Garcia *et al* 1987).

As Inch (1985) points out, controlled cord traction is potentially hazardous for the following reasons:

1. The cord may snap, necessitating operative delivery of the placenta;

2. Pulling on the cord may result in partial detachment of the placenta, leaving behind a cotyledon which may cause haemorrhage or infection;

3. The uterus may be inverted. Kitchen *et al* (1975) quote inversion rates of approximately 1 in 5000 deliveries, and cite Donald (1969) who states 'although inversion may occur spontaneously, mismanagement of the third stage of labour is generally conceded to be the immediate cause'.

Presumably the risks of these hazards would be considerably reduced if the placenta had separated from the wall of the uterus before controlled cord traction. Indeed, some midwives appear to prefer to await signs of separation and descent.

☐ **Awaiting signs of separation and descent**

In a small, local survey of the opinions of midwives regarding their preferred management of the third stage, Levy and Moore (1985) noted that approximately half usually awaited signs of separation and descent before pulling on the cord (despite hospital policy that these signs should *not* be awaited). The signs thought most reliable by the midwives were lengthening of the umbilical cord (after removing any 'slack' of cord from the vagina – application of a clamp to the cord near the vagina facilitated recognition of this sign), and a small trickle of blood per vaginam.

Levy and Moore studied the management of the third stages of 489 women delivered normally. They found that waiting for placental separation increased the mean length of the third stage by approximately one minute. The postpartum haemorrhage rate was significantly higher at 15 per cent when the midwife unsuccessfully attempted 'immediate' controlled cord traction (that is to say, without waiting for signs of separation and descent apart from contraction of the uterus), and then waited for a few minutes before reapplying controlled cord traction. Postpartum haemorrhage rates were similar (about 5 per cent) in the group in which signs were awaited and that in which 'immediate' controlled cord traction was successful at the first attempt.

Levy and Moore suggested that in the two latter groups of women placental separation was at least almost complete when the midwife pulled on the cord and so the placenta was easily delivered. However, in the group where 'immediate' controlled cord traction failed, the placenta may have still been too firmly attached to the uterine wall; the midwife may have merely succeeded in interfering with uterine action and the natural process of separation by pulling on the cord, thus causing increased blood loss from a partially separated placenta.

It is the partially separated placenta that causes bleeding, and once controlled cord traction is initiated it is probably advisable to continue the traction until the placenta is delivered. But there are occasions when controlled cord traction may need to be interrupted for a few minutes. A common example is when the cord starts to tear; the remaining cord is usually inaccessibly high in the vagina or in the uterus, and the midwife then has to employ other techniques, such as maternal effort or fundal pressure to achieve delivery. If these fail (perhaps because the lower segment has by then contracted under the influence of ergometrine), then the length of the third stage extends and the risks of haemorrhage and the need for manual removal increase. By discontinuing controlled cord traction, however, the placenta can then be allowed 'naturally' to separate sufficiently for gently reapplied controlled cord traction to succeed.

Levy and Moore consequently advocate waiting for signs of placental separation and descent prior to controlled cord traction. This was, however, a small study and methodological problems were not wholly resolved. A further, more rigorously controlled, study is needed to assess the benefits of awaiting signs of placental separation and descent before pulling on the cord.

■ Factors predisposing to postpartum haemorrhage

Midwifery and obstetric textbooks cite lists of factors which are thought to predispose to postpartum haemorrhage. These lists include previous third stage problems, overdistension of the uterus by polyhydramnios or multiple pregnancy, antepartum haemorrhage, prolonged or rapid labour, certain anaesthetic drugs, fibroids, grandmultiparity, mismanagement by undue interference with the uterus, full bladder, partially separated placenta, retained blood clot or placental tissue, trauma, inverted uterus and coagulation failures.

The relationship of some of these factors to postpartum haemorrhage may require reassessment especially in the light of changing socioeconomic factors, as the association may no longer be as well established as previously thought. For example, although some studies (Al-Sibai *et al* 1987; Henson *et al* 1987) report a greater incidence of postpartum haemorrhage in grandmultiparae, others (Eidelman *et al* 1988; Seidman *et al* 1988) have found no such association. Eidelman and colleagues argue that grandmultiparity in itself is not a risk factor to postpartum haemorrhage but that previous reports may have reflected the effects of social class rather than parity.

Recent investigation has identified other risk factors for postpartum haemorrhage. For example, the results of a retrospective study of 1000 consecutive deliveries (Brinsden & Clarke 1978) indicate that postpartum haemorrhage is significantly associated with induction of labour by amniotomy and intravenous oxytocin, particularly in primiparous mothers. The indications for induction are not specified in this or similar studies; this information may be relevant as it might be the underlying obstetric problem requiring induction rather than the induction itself that results in haemorrhage.

Brinsden and Clarke suggest that induced labour is shorter and more intense than spontaneous labour, that the uterus becomes 'tired' after delivery, and consequently does not contract and retract efficiently. Furthermore, they consider that if the uterus has been exposed to high doses of oxytocics during the preceeding hours, then it is less likely to respond to a bolus dose of Syntometrine. They also consider the incidence of cervical and vaginal tears is greater when labour is induced.

Hall *et al* (1985) carried out a retrospective study of over 36 000 women delivered normally of singletons between 1967 and 1981. They found the incidence of retained placenta had remained steady at approximately two per cent throughout the 14 years of the study period. The incidence of postpartum haemorrhage showed a marked increase during this period, and was much higher when retained placenta was present (21 per cent as against 3.5 per cent). Hall considered the apparent rise in the postpartum haemorrhage rate may have reflected changing policies regarding the measurement and recording of blood loss (the volume of blood loss had only been recorded since 1976).

Postpartum haemorrhage was significantly more common in primiparae, and also when labour had been induced: the latter association was present both in induced primiparae and multiparae. The increased prevalence of primiparae, and a rise in the induction rate, may also have affected the postpartum haemorrhage rate.

There was no significant association between retained placenta and parity, or induction of labour. Third stage complications tended to recur: the risk was increased threefold (or more if induction of labour was performed) after a previous abnormal third stage.

In a retrospective survey of 489 normal singleton deliveries, Moore and Levy (1982) found postpartum haemorrhage to be significantly associated with induction of labour by amniotomy alone or together with intravenous oxytocin, and with acceleration of labour by intravenous oxytocin. They also found a highly significant association between postpartum haemorrhage and third stages lasting longer than 18 minutes and this accords with other studies which have noted higher postpartum haemorrhage rates when retained placenta is present. Moore and Levy failed to find any significant association between postpartum haemorrhage and maternal age, parity, lengths of first and second stages, gestational age, or birthweight of the baby.

Gilbert *et al* (1987) have noted the apparent increase in postpartum haemorrhage rates over past years and considered that changes in obstetric practice may be responsible for this increase. They compared labour characteristics in 86 women who had a postpartum haemorrhage of more than 500 ml with 351 women whose blood loss at delivery was less than 350 ml. Women with an intermediate blood loss were excluded from the study in order to facilitate a clear definition between the postpartum haemorrhage and non-postpartum haemorrhage groups. All women had prophylactic Syntometrine except those who were hypertensive who were given oxytocin alone. Some women had the conventional active management of the third stage, others requested late clamping of the cord and spontaneous expulsion of the placenta.

Gilbert and colleagues found significant associations between postpartum haemorrhage and primiparity, and induction of labour by amniotomy and intravenous oxytocin (even when the influence of higher forceps rates in primiparae and women with induced labours was excluded). Significant associations were also found between haemorrhage and longer first and second stages even when normal deliveries were achieved, (it appeared that the total length of the second stage was the influential factor, not just the length of pushing), forceps deliveries (both rotational and non-rotational), and the administration of prophylactic oxytocin instead of Syntometrine.

Gilbert and her colleagues found no association between postpartum haemorrhage and maternal age nor, surprisingly, the length of the third stage (although they did not specify the lengths of the third stages); nor did they find that controlled cord traction was associated with less haemorrhage. A weak association was identified between postpartum haemorrhage and birthweight, but in which direction is not specified.

It has been suggested that there is a higher blood loss when the mother adopts an upright position for delivery. In a randomised controlled trial (Stewart *et al* 1983) of 189 deliveries allocated to either a delivery bed or a birthing chair the overall blood loss was found to be greater in the chair. The authors considered that this might be explained by the observation that some multiparae had very rapid deliveries in the upright position and these were associated with haemorrhage from an atonic uterus; similarly, rapid deliveries in the dorsal position did not show this association. Perineal lacerations also seemed to bleed more profusely in the upright position: venous pressure would have been increased in the perineal area and was thought to be the probable cause. Thirdly, (but this was thought to have been of minimal importance) not so many drapes were used and more blood drained into the receptacle and was consequently more accurately estimated.

These findings were supported by another randomised controlled trial (Turner *et al* 1986) in which 636 mothers were allocated to either the standard delivery bed or the Birth EZ chair (tilted back to an angle of 40 degrees) for the second and third stages of labour. Mothers delivered in the chair were significantly more likely to experience postpartum haemorrhage (8.8 per cent as against 3.7 per cent – $p = 0.02$).

In summary, recent studies have indicated that the following factors are associated with higher blood loss in the third stage:

● Primiparity;

● Induction of labour;

● Longer labours;

● Forceps deliveries;

● Previous third stage abnormalities;

● retained placenta;

● delivering in the upright position.

Some of these predisposing factors are rarely mentioned in textbooks. Other risk factors may remain to be identified; for instance, Goodfellow *et al* (1983) found epidural analgesia to be associated with a reduction in plasma oxytocin values during the second stage of labour.

Further research is needed to establish the degree of risk which other traditionally cited factors do in reality confer.

☐ **Estimation of blood loss**

Research into the management of the third stage of labour is complicated by the many variables that may influence the execution of the study and analysis of the data. For example, the volume of blood lost is a vital parameter in assessing the management of the third stage.

The primary danger of the third stage is that of haemorrhage; blood is lost from the placental site and/or from traumatised tissue, such as a torn perineum. 'Traumatic' haemorrhage is often more readily diagnosed; if the uterus is felt to be contracted then the placental site is unlikely to be the source of the haemorrhage. Furthermore, tissue damage, and often the damaged blood vessels themselves, are frequently visible. 'Traumatic' haemorrhage usually responds readily to treatment. It is haemorrhage from the placental site that tends to pose more risk to the mother.

All studies comparing third stage blood loss with another variable are complicated by the problems inherent in accurately measuring blood loss. In many cases, the amount is probably underestimated, particularly when major losses are considered. Blood clots; it soaks into drapes and pads and drips onto the floor; it may or may not be mixed with amniotic fluid. These factors hinder accurate assessment of the quantity of blood lost. Brant (1967) calculated that the true postpartum haemorrhage rate (500 ml or over) is probably about 20 per cent. He calculated the blood loss at 57 deliveries by using a spectrometer to measure the oxyhaemoglobin of the blood loss and calculated this against the mother's total fluid loss and venous haemoglobin at delivery. He noted that amounts of blood loss up to 300 ml were accurately estimated, but above this figure underestimation became more likely; the higher the blood loss, the greater the underestimation.

Levy and Moore (1985) conducted a small experiment to assess the accuracy of blood loss estimation. Four units of date-expired blood were measured into four different amounts (100 ml, 300 ml, 500 ml and 1200 ml); 200 ml of normal saline were added to each amount to mimic a 'moderate' amount of amniotic fluid. Each of the four measured amounts of

Table 7.1 Results of blood loss estimation experiment (all figures given in mls)

Amount of blood	Variation in estimation	Mode	Mean	Error in estimation
100	20–400	100	111	+11
300	65–550	200	197	−103
500	125–750	250	307	−193
1200	450–2000	550	718	−482

blood were assigned to a trolley, set up as though a delivery had taken place. Some of the blood and saline mixture was poured onto the drapes and pads, and the remainder was left in a jug on each trolley. Participants were then invited to estimate the total blood loss on each of the four trolleys.

The results of this experiment (see Table 7.1) confirmed Brant's findings that volumes of blood up to 300 ml are accurately estimated, and that the higher the loss the greater the underestimation. This finding also supported Haswell's (1981) study in which he found that losses over 500 ml were on average underestimated by about a half.

It is likely that most obstetric units employ a policy of using central venous pressure monitoring in cases of major postpartum haemorrhage in order to ensure that the amount of blood replaced is appropriate. However, for 'intermediate' haemorrhages (up to perhaps 1000 ml) when central venous pressure lines are not so likely to be used, perhaps it needs to be born in mind that the true blood loss may be double the estimated amount.

■ Clamping the cord

This chapter has been concerned with maternal aspects of the third stage and will not address any aspect of neonatal management, apart from that of the timing of cord clamping.

Inch (1985) writes, 'If an oxytocic agent is given, the midwife has to decide between clamping the cord immediately the baby is born, thereby denying him his extra physiological quota of blood, or alternatively leaving the cord and risking the probability of a substantial over-transfusion as blood is forced along the cord by the pharmacologically energised contractions of the uterus'.

The blood volume of a newborn infant may vary between 77 ml/kg to 120 ml/kg, depending on whether clamping of the cord has been performed early, or delayed until three minutes or more after birth (Oh *et al* 1966). Suggestions that the extra transfusion associated with late clamping may overload the infant's cardiovascular system are borne out by Yao and Lind

(1977) who, in a study of 13 normal full term infants, found that late cord clamping significantly affected left ventricular performance. Yao and Lind point out that 'in no other situation in life does this physiologic phenomena occur in such an abrupt manner that a transfusion of as much as 100 ml of blood can occur within 3 minutes to a 3 Kg infant' and further note that the blood volume of an 'early clamped' infant is approximately that of the fetus at term. They nevertheless consider that normal babies are probably able to adapt to the increased blood volume although Hohmann (1985) recommends that following normal deliveries the cord should be clamped after one or two minutes.

There is some evidence that preterm babies deprived of this transfusion experience higher rates of respiratory distress syndrome. Hohmann (1985) suggests that late cord clamping may be advantageous to preterm infants as the incidence of respiratory distress syndrome is reduced with late clamping and subsequent increased transfusion of blood. He points out that, if intra-uterine hypoxia has occurred, increased placental transfusion will already have taken place *in utero* to improve the oxygenation of the fetus, and cord clamping and resuscitation can proceed immediately after delivery.

The extra transfusion of blood in 'late clamped' infants may predispose towards physiological jaundice. Prendiville *et al* (1988b), in their controlled trial of 'active' versus 'physiological' management of the third stage, did indeed find more neonatal jaundice in the group of babies whose cords were clamped late. Moss and Monset-Couchard (1967) in a review of 10 studies, failed to find a conclusive link between late cord clamping and neonatal jaundice in normal babies, although they noted raised serum bilirubin levels in a small group of preterm babies.

It is possible that early clamping of the cord predisposes to feto-maternal transfusion because of the increased back-pressure of blood within the cord; this has obvious implications when considering, for example, sensitisation of the rhesus negative woman delivered of a rhesus positive baby. In a study of 200 normal deliveries, Lapido (1972) did indeed find a significantly greater incidence of feto-maternal transfusion when the cord was clamped at delivery than when free bleeding of the placental end of the cord was allowed, or when cessation of cord pulsation was awaited before clamping. He therefore advocated the practice of late cord clamping as an additional safeguard to Anti-D prophylaxis in the prevention of iso-immunisation.

■ Implications of research findings

The policy of 'active' management of the third stage of labour appears to be justified in terms of reducing blood loss at delivery. Active management implies firstly the administration of an oxytocic – ideally Syntometrine (unless the mother is hypertensive), as this oxytocic is associated with less blood loss than other oxytocics.

But what constitutes an 'acceptable' blood loss? What are the actual effects of postpartum haemorrhage in terms of, for example, tiredness, lactation or puerperal infection? Postpartum haemorrhage is defined as a blood loss of 500 ml or over, or any amount sufficient to adversely affect the mother. However, if a mother enters labour in normal health and with an adequate haemoglobin, then she is unlikely to be adversely affected by a blood loss of 500 ml. The defined amount of blood loss constituting postpartum haemorrhage may therefore need upward redefinition.

Blood is arguably the world's most precious commodity. To women in underdeveloped countries it is particularly precious and whatever measures their birth attendants take to prevent blood loss are almost certainly justified. But oxytocics have been shown to have side effects such as nausea, vomiting and headache. Can we really justify imposing these symptoms on a healthy woman merely in order to save her an extra few hundred millilitres of blood?

As well as implying the prophylactic use of oxytocics, active management also involves controlled cord traction, usually as soon as the uterus has contracted. There may well be merit in awaiting signs of separation as the study by Levy and Moore (1985) suggests, although further studies need to be undertaken into this aspect of management.

What really does place a mother at increased risk of haemorrhage? What degree of risk do the traditionally quoted predisposing factors actually confer upon the mother, in view of current obstetric practices and (probably even more relevant) women's relatively higher standards of nutrition and general health?

Are there circumstances when we need to adapt our management of the third stage, or is one (fairly rigidly defined) method appropriate for every mother? If not, what are these circumstances, and what aspect of our management should then be changed? Randomised controlled trials are needed.

Midwives conduct the vast majority of third stages; we need to find the answers to these questions for it is around them that our present practice revolves.

■ Recommendations for clinical practice in the light of currently available evidence

In the management of the third stage of labour, consideration should be given to the following points.

1. Syntometrine is the oxytocic of choice, except when the mother is hypertensive when oxytocin alone may be more appropriate.

2. Active management of the third stage appears to be justified in terms of reducing blood loss.

3. Signs of placental separation and descent should be awaited prior to controlled cord traction. Suggested signs (in addition to contraction of the uterus) are cord lengthening and a trickle of blood per vaginam.

4. If 'physiological' management is attempted but active intervention needed, then management must proceed actively.

5. Blood losses estimated at over 500 ml may need to be doubled in order to reach a more accurate estimation.

6. Primiparity, induction of labour, delivering in an upright position, and forceps delivery appear to be predisposing factors to postpartum haemorrhage.

7. There *may* be benefits in late clamping of the cord, especially in the case of women at risk of iso-immunisation, or in preterm deliveries where the baby does not need immediate resuscitation.

■ Practice check

- What factors do you take into consideration when deciding upon your method of third stage management?

- How many mothers in your care delivered 'actively' of their placenta remember the third stage of labour, and what are their comments regarding this stage?

- Do you ever conduct 'physiological' third stages? If not, why?

- If you would like to conduct 'physiological' third stages but feel you do not have enough experience or confidence, could your midwifery manager or Supervisor of Midwives help you in this respect?

- What is the postpartum haemorrhage rate in your unit?

- From your unit's records, can you identify factors that appear to be associated with postpartum haemorrhage?

- What is the postpartum haemorrhage rate associated with *your* deliveries?

- Ask a colleague who has assisted you at a delivery for her estimation of total blood loss. How closely does this agree with your estimation (in total honesty)?

- From your observation of newly delivered mothers, what effect does postpartum haemorrhage appear to have on their postnatal progress?

- How many mothers require readmission for removal of retained products of conception? Is there any indication in these mother's records that the placenta or membranes were delivered incomplete?

■ References

Al-Sibai M H, Rahman M S, Rahman J 1987 Obstetric problems in the grand-multipara – a clinical study of 1330 cases. Journal of Obstetrics and Gynaecology 8: 135–138

Brant H A 1967 Precise estimation of postpartum haemorrhage: difficulties and importance. British Medical Journal 1: 398–400

Brinsden P R S, Clark A D 1978 Postpartum haemorrhage after induced and spontaneous labour. British Medical Journal 2: 855–56

DHSS 1989 Confidential enquiries into maternal deaths in England and Wales. HMSO, London

Donald I 1969 Practical obstetric problems, 4th ed: 731–37. Lloyd-Luke, London

Eidelman A I, Kamar R, Schimmel M S, Bar-On E 1988 The grandmultipara – is she still a risk? American Journal of Obstetrics and Gynecology 158: 389–92

Embrey M P, Barber D T C, Scudamore J H 1963 Use of Syntometrine in prevention of postpartum haemorrhage. British Medical Journal 1: 1387–89

Elbourne D, Prendiville W, Chalmers I 1988 Choice of oxytocic preparation for routine use in the management of the third stage of labour: an overview of the evidence from controlled trials. British Journal of Obstetrics and Gynaecology 95: 17–30

Garcia J, Garforth S, Ayers S 1987 The policy and practice of midwifery study: introduction and methods. Midwifery 3: 2–9

Gilbert L, Porter W, Brown V A 1987 Postpartum haemorrhage – a continuing problem. British Journal of Obstetrics and Gynaecology 94: 67–71

Goodfellow C F, Hull M G R, Swaab D F, Dogterom J, Buijs R M 1983 Oxytocin deficiency at delivery with epidural analgesia. British Journal of Obstetrics and Gynaecology 90: 214–19

Hall M H, Halliwell R, Carr-Hill R 1985 Concomitant and repeated happenings of complications of the third stage of labour. British Journal of Obstetrics and Gynaecology 92: 732–38

Harding J E 1988 Problems experienced when running a large randomised controlled trial MIDIRS (Midwives Information and Resource Service), Information Pack No 7

Haswell J N 1981 Measured blood loss at delivery. Journal of Indiana State Medical Association 74(1): 34–6

Henson G L, Knott P D, Colley N V 1987 The dangerous multipara – fact or fiction? Journal of Obstetrics and Gynaecology 8: 130–34

Hibbard B M 1964 The third stage of labour. British Medical Journal 1: 1485–88

Hohmann M 1985 Early or late cord clamping? A question of optimal time. Wiener Klinische Wochenschrift 97(11): 497–500

Inch S 1983 Third stage management. Association of Radical Midwives Newsletter 19 (Autumn)

Inch S 1985 Management of the third stage of labour – another cascade of intervention? Midwifery 1: 114–22

Kitchen J D, Thiagarajah S, May H V, Thornton W N 1975 Puerperal inversion of the uterus. American Journal of Obstetrics and Gynecology 1: 51–8

Lapido O A 1972 Management of third stage of labour, with particular reference to reduction of feto-maternal transfusion. British Medical Journal 1: 721–23

Levy V A, Moore J V 1985 The midwife's management of the third stage of labour. Nursing Times 81(39): 47–50

Milner I 1989 Personal communication

Moore J V, Levy V A 1982 Further research into the management of the third stage of labour and the incidence of postpartum haemorrhage. In Research and the Midwife Conference Proceedings: 106–11. Available from the University of Manchester, Department of Nursing Studies

Moss A J, Monset-Couchard M 1967 Placental transfusion: early versus late clamping of the umbilical cord. Paediatrics 40: 109–26

Oh W, Blankenship W, Lind J 1966 Further study of neonatal blood volume in relation to placental transfusion. Annales Paediatrici (Basel) 207: 147–59

Prendiville W, Elbourne D, Chalmers I 1988a The effects of routine oxytocic administration in the management of the third stage of labour: an overview of the evidence from controlled trials. British Journal of Obstetrics and Gynaecology 95: 3–16

Prendiville W J, Harding J E, Elbourne D R, Stirrat G M 1988b The Bristol third stage trial: active versus physiological management of third stage of labour. British Medical Journal 297: 1295–1300

Seideman D S, Arman Y, Roll D, Stevenson D K, Gale R 1988 Grand multiparity: an obstetric or neonatal risk factor? American Journal of Obstetrics and Gynecology 158: 1034–39

Spencer P M 1962 Controlled cord traction in management of the third stage of labour. British Medical Journal II: 1728–32

Sorbe B 1978 Active pharmacological management of the third stage of labour. Obstetrics and Gynaecology 52: 694–97

Stewart P, Hillan E, Calder A A 1983 A randomised trial to evaluate the use of a birth chair for delivery. Lancet ii: 1296–98

Turner M J, Romney M L, Webb J B, Gordon H 1986 The birthing chair: an obstetric hazard? Journal of Obstetrics and Gynaecology 6: 232–35

Yao A C, Lind J 1977 Effect of early and late cord clamping on the systolic time intervals of the newborn infant. Acta Paediatrica Scandinavica 66: 489–93

■ Suggested further reading

Prendiville W, Elbourne D R 1989 The third stage of labour. In Chalmers I, Enkins M, Keirse M (eds) Effective care in pregnancy and childbirth. Oxford University Press, Oxford

Chapter 8

HIV infection – a midwifery perspective

Carolyn Roth and Janette Brierley

Currently only a small portion of those in Britain infected with the Human Immunodeficiency Virus (HIV) are female, but the incidence of infection among women is rising and many are of childbearing age (Chin 1988). Inevitably an increasing number of women will present in pregnancy with known HIV infection or will request HIV antibody testing which subsequently proves positive. Midwives must acquire the knowledge and skills to give care which is sensitive to and protects the interests of these women.

Many women with HIV infection will come from a background of injecting drug use and multiple social deprivation, and this must be taken into consideration when planning care. In addition, enormous social stigma surrounds HIV disease and once it has been diagnosed it will have an irrevocable impact on a woman's life. This chapter will examine some of the clinical, professional and ethical considerations involved in developing a midwifery response to the challenge of HIV infection.

■ **It is assumed that you are already aware of the following:**

- The physical characteristics of the Human Immunodeficiency Virus;

- How it is spread between adults;

- The length of the period of seroconversion (i.e. the time between becoming infected and producing antibodies to the virus);

- The social and psychological implications of being HIV antibody positive;

154

- The incubation period of the infection (i.e. the time between becoming infected and becoming ill);

- The physical effects of HIV infection in adults.

■ HIV and the health care worker

An important obstacle to the provision of appropriate care to women and babies who may be infected by HIV is the uncertainty and fear among health workers about their risk of acquiring this serious infection in the course of delivering care.

Data which has been gathered since the advent of the HIV epidemic indicates that the risk of accidental exposure to HIV in a health care setting is very small. The world literature reports only 35 cases of health care workers infected by HIV as a result of occupational exposure (Gill & Porter 1989). There have been a number of prospective and cross-sectional studies following up health care workers who have experienced inoculation of infected blood as a result of percutaneous injury (broken skin). These studies have so far followed up 1852 exposures to infected blood. Amongst these, six individuals became HIV positive, and an additional three were presumed to be infected. The risk of infection following inoculation by infected blood is therefore calculated as 0.49 per cent.

Nineteen health care workers (some of whom appear amongst those referred to above) have become HIV positive after a specific exposure to infected blood, and of these 14 were exposed as the result of needlestick or other sharps injury. The remaining five reported heavy or prolonged skin, mucous membrane and/or conjunctival exposure to blood (Henderson 1988; Gill & Porter 1989). A further 13 health care workers infected with HIV are presumed to have been infected as the result of occupational exposure. Eight additional surveys have been conducted on a total of 2 957 health care workers, many of them caring for individuals known to be infected by HIV. Of those surveyed, three individuals were found to be infected with HIV, but in only one could infection be linked to occupational exposure. This was a dentist who did not routinely wear gloves and who acknowledged 10 percutaneous injuries in the previous five years (Henderson 1988).

Serological surveys of more than 700 household contacts of individuals infected with HIV, including one survey of boys sharing accommodation at boarding school (Berthier *et al* 1986), have failed to provide any evidence for transmission of HIV infection except to the sexual partners of infected individuals or to children born to infected mothers (Henderson 1988). The small risk of health workers being accidentally exposed to infection by HIV is specifically related to sharps injuries, or prolonged or extensive skin or mucous membrane exposure to blood.

■ Implications of HIV infection for pregnant women and their babies

□ What effect does pregnancy have on the health of the HIV infected woman?

The theoretical possibility that the immunosuppressive effect of pregnancy might combine with that of HIV disease and give rise to a worsening prognosis has been of great concern (Schoenbaum *et al* 1988). This concern seemed to be confirmed by a number of studies conducted early in the epidemic which demonstrated a worsened prognosis for women with HIV infection, apparently as a consequence of pregnancy (Scott *et al* 1985; Minkoff *et al* 1987). The women followed in these studies, however, were selected retrospectively on the basis of having previously given birth to infants who developed AIDS or other HIV-related illness. This may have biased the sample towards women who were at a more advanced stage of infection at the time of the subsequent pregnancy.

Prospective studies of HIV antibody positive women in Scotland and France did not demonstrate any adverse effect on their clinical or immunological status as a consequence of pregnancy (Berrebi *et al* 1988; MacCallum *et al* 1988). Three out of 35 (9 per cent) of the HIV seropositive women followed in a West German study, however, although well during pregnancy, experienced clinical progression of illness as well as deterioration of immunological status postnatally (Schaefer *et al* 1988). A recent American study of 102 pregnant women at high risk of HIV infection reported a decline in immune indices in the 37 HIV-positive women. This was more marked during pregnancy than postnatally and was at a faster rate than that observed in HIV-infected homosexual men and haemophiliacs in other studies. It is suggested that this may be evidence of acceleration in pregnancy of the immunosuppression associated with HIV infection (Biggar *et al* 1989). The evidence so far available is insufficient to provide a conclusive answer as to the effect of pregnancy on HIV disease, and there is clearly an urgent need for well-designed studies to investigate this. Such studies would compare the course of HIV infection in a group of pregnant woman with its course in a matched group of non-pregnant controls.

□ What effect does HIV infection have on the progress and outcome of pregnancy?

Data providing answers to this question are also limited but no evidence has emerged to suggest that HIV infection in itself has an adverse effect on pregnancy outcome.

A study in Scotland comparing the pregnancies of asymptomatic, HIV-positive pregnant women with those of HIV-negative women showed no differences in maternal pregnancy complications, mean birth weight, gestational age, perinatal mortality or fetal abnormality. The spontaneous abortion rate however was higher in the HIV infected women. The high rate of prematurity and intrauterine growth retardation in both groups reflected the background of social deprivation and lifestyle common to the women, all of whom had either been intravenous drug users or had had seropositive partners (Johnstone *et al* 1988). A large prospective study in Kinshasa, Zaire has not demonstrated an increased risk of spontaneous abortion or stillbirth in 479 HIV-seropositive women compared with 583 HIV-seronegative women matched for age and parity (Nsa *et al* 1988).

☐ **What effect does maternal HIV infection have on the health of the fetus/neonate?**

Transmission of HIV from mother to fetus certainly occurs, though the exact route of infection is difficult to confirm, and why it occurs in some cases and not in others is not clear.

■ Routes of transmission

☐ *In utero*/transplacental transmission

There is substantial evidence that HIV is transmitted to the fetus *in utero*. HIV has been isolated from fetal tissue in a pregnancy terminated at 20 weeks gestation with intact membrances (Jovaisas *et al* 1986). The virus has also been cultured from amniotic fluid and placental tissue (Sprecher *et al* 1986). HIV was cultured from the cord blood of 22 infants (23 per cent) of 94 HIV-seropositive women enrolled in a study in Zaire (Ryder *et al* 1988).

☐ Transmission at delivery

HIV has been found in cervical secretions (Vogt *et al* 1986), and is present in the blood of an infected mother, to which the newborn is exposed at the time of birth regardless of the route of delivery. A small study (Semprini *et al* 1986) which compared vaginal and caesarean delivery failed to demonstrate any difference in the rate of infection to the infant. Infection at the time of delivery is *theoretically* possible, but methods of confirming this route of transmission are not available and it is thus impossible to determine what contribution this makes to neonatal infection rates.

□ **Postnatal transmission via breast milk**

HIV has been isolated from the breast milk of asymptomatic HIV antibody positive women (Thiry *et al* 1985). In addition, there have now been eight case reports of women who became infected with HIV early in the postnatal period (six of them as a consequence of a seropositive blood transfusion), whose breastfeeding babies also seroconverted, presumably because of infected breastmilk (Ryder & Hassig 1988). These reports clearly demonstrate a risk of this route of transmission, but it is impossible to calculate its contribution to perinatal infection and whether it represents an increased risk to the neonate who was exposed to HIV during the course of the pregnancy. The answer to that question will only emerge from follow up of the babies of HIV positive mothers and comparison of infection rates according to feeding practice. Another important, but as yet unresearched, area is that of the benefits that breastfeeding might confer on the potentially immunocompromised HIV infected baby (WHO 1987; Minchin, 1988).

■ **Rate of transmission to the neonate**

Follow up of the infants of HIV infected mothers has produced a wide range of incidence of infection depending on the population studied and the length of follow up. In one study of 20 women who had previously delivered one infant who had developed AIDS, 65 per cent of the infants in subsequent pregnancies were infected (Schoenbaum 1988). Preliminary figures from the multicentred European study which is prospectively following up the infants of HIV positive women, so far indicate a transmission rate of 24 per cent (Peckham *et al* 1988). Figures from Kinshasa demonstrate markedly different neonatal infection rates in the babies of two groups of HIV infected women. Transmission to the babies of women of lower socio-economic status, who had a greater incidence of symptomatic infection, was 65 per cent while in the babies of better off, asymptomatic women the rate was about 30 per cent. (Ryder & Hassig 1988). Such disparate findings probably reflect different stages of maternal illness in a particular population. It seems probable, therefore, that rates of maternal-neonatal transmission may change over time as infection within the population becomes established, and this makes it difficult to predict transmission rates with any certainty.

Diagnosis of HIV infection in the neonate is problematic. All babies of HIV positive mothers will be born with passively acquired maternal antibody, and this may persist for as long as 18 months. In addition, some babies who become HIV antibody negative nonetheless may be infected with the virus (Peckham *et al* 1988).

Confirmation of infection may be achieved by detection of p24 antigen, but this requires a quantity of serum which is difficult to obtain. Newer laboratory techniques involving amplification of DNA are being developed and will improve the prospects of early diagnosis of HIV infection in the baby of an infected mother (Peckham *et al* 1988). Recent work on the detection of I_gA HIV antibodies suggests that, combined with clinical information on an infant, this may be an effective method for the early diagnosis of HIV infection in asymptomatic infants (Weiblen *et al* 1990).

☐ The presentation of infection in the infant

Signs of HIV infection are rarely detected at birth but the majority of infected children present initially with nonspecific signs and symptoms such as recurrent respiratory infections, recurrent diarrhoea, unexplained fevers, recurrent oral thrush and failure to thrive. Other findings include persistent generalised lymphadenopathy, persistent hepatomegaly or splenomegaly, lymphocytic interstitial pneumonitis, acquired microcephaly and failure to reach or regression from developmental milestones. Prospective studies are following up the course of infection in those children who remain healthy carriers and those whose infection status is indeterminant (Rubenstein & Bernstein 1986; Mok 1988; Peckham *et al* 1988; Mok 1989).

☐ HIV infection: the midwifery response

Our response to the challenge of HIV infection in maternity care must take account of several areas of concern:

- The implications of this blood-borne virus for clinical practice, taking into account how we should adapt our practice in order to reduce to the minimum any risk of exposure to care givers;
- The effect of the virus on the health of infected women and their babies;
- The need to develop care in a way which protects women and babies from the stigma of HIV infection and which offers them a positive contribution towards their future.

■ Infection control policies

It is essential that midwives and other clinicians develop and maintain high standards of hygiene and safety in their clinical practice to minimise the small risk of accidental exposure occurring. Particular attention should be paid to practices which involve possible contact with blood and other potentially infectious body fluids and to procedures where accidental sharps injury might occur.

Policies which aim to limit the risks of HIV exposure must be applied in *all* clinical situations and their application should not depend on knowledge of the HIV status of the individual (Morbidity & Mortality Weekly Report 1987). In this way, a safe standard of practice will be applied in the care of all women – those known to be infected with HIV, those who have not been tested, and those who are infected but have had a negative test result initially because they have not yet seroconverted.

The following principles of safe practice have been suggested (Morbidity & Mortality Weekly Report 1987, 1988).

1. Care must be taken to *prevent injuries* when using, cleaning or disposing of sharp instruments or equipment.

2. *Protective barriers* should be used to prevent skin and mucous membrane exposure to blood, body fluids which contain visible blood, as well as certain other body fluids including vaginal secretions, cerebrospinal fluid and amniotic fluid; (we have named only those with a direct relevance for midwifery practice.) Precautions are not required for contact with breast milk, although where contact is frequent, for example in milk banks, gloves should be worn. The type of barrier(s) used should be appropriate to the procedure being performed and the exposure anticipated.

3. Hands and other skin surfaces which have been contaminated with blood or other body fluids to which precautions apply, should be washed with soap and water thoroughly and immediately.

Policies should be consistent and as simple to apply as possible. It may be useful to produce a list of ground rules for use within a particular unit, which would include those listed below.

1. Cuts or lesions on the hands should be covered by waterproof plasters.

2. Gloves must be worn during all procedures in which contact with blood, liquor or vaginal secretions may occur.

3. Needles must never be resheathed and must be disposed of immediately in an approved container.

4. When extensive contamination is anticipated, as at the time of artificial rupture of membranes or at delivery, a waterproof apron covered by a protective gown or a water repellent gown should be worn. The use of eye protection and masks has been recommended because of the possibility of transmission of virus through

conjunctival or mucous membrane exposure due to splashing. Spectacles can be used for eye protection and are preferable to goggles and visors, because they are less obtrusive.

5. If a sharps injury does occur or there is accidental exposure of the skin, the area should immediately be washed with soap and water. *If there has been a puncture wound, free bleeding should be encouraged but the wound should not be sucked* (Department of Health 1990). Eyewash solution, which should be readily available in relevant clinical areas, should be used if eyes have been splashed. The incident should then be reported in accordance with unit policy.

6. All linen soiled with blood or body fluid should be disposed of in a water soluble bag, placed within a red bag. Gloves should be worn when handling fouled linen (RCN 1988).

7. Spillages of blood or liquor should be attended to promptly using a sodium hypochlorite (bleach) solution in a concentration of 1:100 to 1:10, depending on the amount of material on the surface to be cleaned and disinfected. (Morbidity & Mortality Weekly Report 1987).

■ Considerations for antenatal care

Health promotion and education are components of midwifery practice which offer an ideal opportunity for preventive education about HIV. Midwives meet all women who attend for antenatal care and are often in the privileged position of learning about a woman's lifestyle and concerns about her sexual life. This places midwives in a particularly favourable position to inform and educate about the sexual spread of HIV and, if it is relevant, the hazards of shared needles and syringes.

Making the most of these educational opportunities will require updating of knowledge, the development of effective techniques of teaching and counselling, and nonjudgemental attitudes towards women who might be infected by HIV. The approach to all women must be one of tolerance and respect for without this it is impossible to provide them with information or offer them care.

During history taking at the booking clinic is the most likely time for issues to be raised about high risk experience or behaviour and discussion may elicit factors such as:

● Past or current injecting drug use by a woman and/or her partner;

● Blood transfusion in the UK prior to October 1985 (when screening of blood supplies was introduced), or transfusion in countries where blood is not screened for HIV;

- Prostitution;

- Having a sexual relationship in, or with a partner from, an area where HIV infection is endemic;

- Having a sexual partner who has had relationships with other men.

Not all of these 'risk factors' will be known to a woman and some, even if known, will not be disclosed to the midwife. The objective however should be to provide the women with the opportunity to discuss risk if she would like to, and therefore her decision not to disclose information is not a problem. It is also important to recognise that, as the heterosexual incidence of HIV infection increases, identifiable risks such as intravenous drug use or male bisexuality will be less prominent.

If a woman may have been exposed to HIV, or if a risk factor has been identified in her history, then the availability of antibody testing should be brought to her attention. The booking interview, however, may not be the best time to explore the question of possible infection or that of HIV testing, particularly if it is the first time a woman is considering the issue.

☐ **Problems with discussing testing at booking**

1. There is likely to be an 'overload' of other information for the woman to absorb at this visit;

2. It may be difficult for the midwife to broach the subject in a way that will not threaten or offend the women, especially if the grounds for considering her to be at risk relate to her place of origin or her sexual experience;

3. She may feel obliged to accept the test along with 'routine' blood tests;

4. The offer of testing may give rise to unnecessary and unacceptable levels of anxiety;

5. It will probably be difficult for her to make a soundly reasoned decision about testing at such short notice.

Some of these difficulties may be overcome by offering all women information to consider before attendance at the booking clinic. This could cover the following:

- HIV infection and how it is spread;

- The behaviour or experience which may put a woman at risk of infection;

- The effect of HIV infection on a woman during pregnancy and on the baby;

- What HIV testing is and its availability to the pregnant woman.

It is important also to allay any concern that HIV testing may be carried out without the woman's permission or knowledge.

A leaflet, or a prebooking group discussion which cover these points will ensure a wider distribution of the information as well as providing a vehicle for introducing the issue in a way which is not threatening or intrusive. A leaflet sent to the woman before she attends for booking can be read and discussed with her partner and/or others and allows her to take the initiative if she believes that testing would be appropriate for her. A different strategy for education will have to be devised for women who do not read or speak English and thought must be given to developing alternative approaches.

☐ **Testing for HIV antibodies during pregnancy**

There has been a temptation to regard screening for HIV antibodies as another screening test which would be advantageous to all pregnant women (New Scientist 1988). It is however important to realise that testing for HIV antibodies has consequences which are different from most of the 'routine' tests which women might choose to have. The debate surrounding HIV testing in pregnancy has highlighted the issue of gaining 'informed consent' for all blood tests, and practices should be re-examined in light of current UKCC guidelines (UKCC 1987). These advise that nurses, midwives and health visitors who take blood without consent or collude with a doctor in obtaining such specimens expose themselves to the possibility of civil action for damages or criminal charges of assault.

HIV testing should not be offered within a maternity unit unless it can be accompanied by thorough pre- and post-test counselling (Miller 1987). This is, of necessity, time consuming but because of the serious consequences of a positive result it is essential that a woman has the opportunity to consider the matter thoroughly. The aim of testing should be to provide options for women regarding their pregnancy and future plans, and it should *never* be regarded as a mechanism for improved infection control.

Midwifery staff must be prepared adequately for their role if they are to offer pretest counselling. The counselling situation should allow the woman to explore with the midwife a number of issues. The first of these is why she wants to be tested. The second is that she understands the significance of a positive test which is that:

- She has been infected with HIV and may become ill in the future, but that it does not mean that she has AIDS;

- She will always be infected with HIV and therefore will always be able to pass the infection to others through unprotected sexual intercourse or sharing 'works' (needles and syringes used for injecting drugs);

- It is possible that her unborn baby will be infected while *in utero* or at birth and, if infected, the baby may become ill and possibly die.

If the antibody test is negative it probably means that she is not infected with HIV, but if exposure may have occurred within the last three months repeat testing is advisable.

- Although HIV antibody negative, she is still at risk of becoming infected and she should be aware of and avoid risky behaviour.

A further issue that the woman needs to consider is how she will prepare herself for the possibility of a positive result and what impact this may have on her, her partner and other family members. Having an HIV antibody test may prevent her from getting insurance or a mortgage, even if the test result proves negative. She may face difficulties regarding employment and medical and dental care if her test result is positive.

The social stigma, fear and profound psychological consequences associated with a diagnosis of HIV infection require that testing should not be undertaken without full consideration of these factors. A woman will need adequate time for this and may choose to return at a later date for the specimen to be taken. Regardless of her decision about being tested, it is important to reinforce the information relevant to her about reducing the risk of sexual transmission of infection and the hazard of shared needles and syringes.

If a woman chooses to be tested, a critical time for her will be when she is informed of her result, and clear plans should be made at the time of collecting the specimen about when the result will be available and where she will come to receive it. She should consider whether there is a close relative or friend who might accompany her at this time so that support will be readily available. She should however be warned to resist the impulse to discuss having the test with others indiscriminately.

Preservation of confidentiality is of paramount importance and this should apply at all stages of a woman's care, including when she expresses an interest in being tested. Biohazard labelling of blood samples and reference on the request form to the possible diagnosis are undesirable if a name is attached, whereas using the case number or another number to identify the sample would be more satisfactory.

☐ **Subsequent care for the HIV positive woman**

The test result must be conveyed in a place which is private, and by someone who has met the woman before, can spend an adequate period of time and feels confident to be able to review with her the significance of the result. It may be valuable for an HIV counsellor to be available at the time of this interview. A woman's initial response to a positive result is likely to be one of shock and intense emotion (Miller 1987). It is unlikely that she will be able to take in much information, or be able to plan rationally at this time, and so a further appointment should be arranged to take place in the next few days. Giving a positive result late in the week should be avoided, unless some contact with known staff can be made by the woman over the weekend if she feels she needs further explanation.

Before leaving the clinic she should also be given the telephone numbers of community-based support organisations (for example, the Terence Higgins Trust or Positively Women) so that she has a 'lifeline' to reach out to at this highly vulnerable time. To date, there are limited facilities offering support to women and midwives should familiarise themselves with what is available and how it can be reached.

A catastrophic reaction to a positive HIV result may be suicide and where possible the woman should not be on her own in the period immediately after receiving a positive result; it is a great advantage if she has identified in advance someone to whom she can turn to at this time.

One of the first issues she may need to consider is whether she wants to continue the pregnancy. Her decision may be helped by reviewing current information about the risks of transmission to her infant and concerns about her own health. She should not feel pressured to accept a termination of pregnancy but her decision must be based on adequate realistic information. Whatever her decision, the importance of safer sexual practices and the practical issues of infection control need to be addressed such as dealing with blood loss and avoiding the sharing of needles and syringes, if relevant. She is likely to need to discuss worries about infection of her partner and any other children she may have.

☐ **Continuing care during pregnancy**

If she decides to continue her pregnancy, it is vital that continuity of midwifery and obstetric care is arranged. This will give the woman an opportunity to develop a relationship with a small supportive team which can respond to her needs and it minimises the number of people who need to know about her HIV status.

Special consideration must be given to preventing accidental disclosure of her HIV status to her family, friends or other hospital staff. Decisions need to be made about whether and how to document a positive result. The practice of obvious marking of notes with a biohazard label can constitute a breach of confidentiality; likewise writing the HIV test result in a prominent place on hospital notes or anywhere on the notes carried by the woman is unacceptable. HIV status should not be entered into a computer record because information from this is often reproduced and widely distributed.

Discussion should take place with the woman about which hospital staff and other health care workers (for example her GP and health visitor) should be informed of her positive HIV result. If she decides to inform others, she might do this herself or prefer to give permission to the midwife or doctor to do it on her behalf.

Antenatal care should be co-ordinated with that of her HIV disease, and liaison established between all those involved (the clinical immunologist and psychologist for example). Information should be consistent and surveillance of her HIV disease must be arranged.

Currently in the UK most antibody positive women will be well; midwives however must be alert to the possible significance of nonspecific symptoms such as fatigue, weight loss, anorexia, diarrhoea and oral thrush (Minkoff 1987). The woman should be encouraged to report any symptoms so that appropriate investigation and treatment may be started. The requirements of good nutrition, adequate rest and avoidance of infection during pregnancy will be particularly important for the woman with HIV infection, although poor social circumstances may make these objectives difficult to achieve without additional financial and other social support. The midwife should be aware of and help facilitate these. The pregnancy may be complicated by the problem of drug dependency and liaison should be maintained with a drug dependency unit if she is already receiving care from one.

The antenatal period should be used to discuss issues of future concern. Opportunity should be provided to meet with the paediatrician to discuss the risks to the baby and to plan for future surveillance of the baby's health.

Time should be allowed to discuss plans for feeding her baby. For the woman planning to breastfeed, it is important that an opportunity be provided for a full discussion of the available evidence about possible breastmilk transmission and how that affects her plans. A decision not to breastfeed may give rise to additional feelings of loss and guilt and she must have the opportunity to express these. The midwife should explore with her the ways she can achieve close physical contact with her baby in spite of not breastfeeding.

Pregnancy may be stressful for any woman. For the woman with HIV infection this period will be further complicated by isolation, grief, loss of self esteem, guilt and anxiety about her physical health as well as the future health of her child. The midwife's care should aim to identify and ameliorate the impact of these problems.

In preparation for labour, explanation of infection control procedures should be offered to the woman, preferably by the midwife already involved in her care.

■ Considerations for care during labour

It is desirable that a midwife whom the woman already knows is the main care provider. As well as being a source of additional support, this reduces the number of extra staff involved in her care and is a further protection of confidentiality.

As long as membranes remain intact, risk to staff of accidental exposure is minimised and therefore artificial rupture of the membranes should be avoided. In the interest of reducing additional risk of virus transmission to the fetus in labour, invasive procedures such as fetal scalp electrodes and fetal blood sampling should be avoided if possible (Scrimgeour 1988). Conscientious application of the ground rules should be the basis for the care of *all* women in labour (see above pages 159–161). Additional guidelines for care in labour include the following.

1. Care should be taken to avoid splashing of blood when the cord is cut.

2. If resuscitation of a baby is required, mechanical suction apparatus should be used.

3. If a baby is fit and well, it should be bathed on the labour ward soon after delivery, to remove all maternal blood and liquor. To avoid the risk of chilling, bath temperature should be 38°C and care should be taken to warm the room adequately. The midwife should wear gloves and a waterproof gown for this procedure.

4. All placentae should be placed in double plastic bags after examination and disposed of by incineration.

5. Showers should be available to staff on the labour ward and should be used if extensive skin contamination by blood or liquor occurs.

■ Considerations for care during the postnatal period

□ The mother

During the postnatal period the emphasis in the care of *all* women should be on self care facilitated by midwifery teaching and support. Practices which demand unnecessary exposure of the midwife or other care givers to blood or blood stained fluids should be abandoned. High standards of personal hygiene should be encouraged for women and there must be adequate provision of receptacles for the safe disposal of sanitary towels.

Showers, rather than baths, should be preferred in planning and equipping postnatal wards.

High standards of housekeeping and domestic hygiene should be achieved, including frequent wiping of surfaces with warm water and detergent, efficient storage and transport of dirty linen, frequent cleaning of bathrooms and toilets. If surfaces are contaminated with blood or body fluids, hypochlorite solution should be used to disinfect them.

It is not essential that a woman with HIV infection have a single room or separate toilet facilities unless she requests this. If at all possible a midwife already known to the woman should be involved in her ongoing care both in hospital and in the community. Her postnatal hospital stay need not be extended unless she is ill, but it is important to devote adequate time postnatally for discussion of contraception. In addition to the condom, which should be used to reduce the risk of transmission of HIV to her sexual partner, the woman should be encouraged to choose another method of contraception to reduce the risk of unintended pregnancy. Arrangements for follow up surveillance of her general health and immunological status should be made before discharge, including regular cervical screening because of the increased risk of cervical dysplasia in the HIV positive woman (Bradbeer 1987). Before a woman's care is transferred into the community, it is important that she has the opportunity to decide about informing other professionals who will be involved in her care about her HIV status.

☐ **The infant**

Care of all babies should be based on the principles of infection control already outlined. No special precautions are necessary for the care of the baby of an HIV-positive woman.

When the midwife is carrying out cord care, she should wear gloves if there is blood loss from the cord stump. Gloves should also be worn for collection of capillary samples of blood (heel prick) because of the high risk of contamination of hands.

The infant of an HIV positive mother will not require admission to the special care baby unit because of HIV, but drug withdrawal may be a complicating feature. If this is anticipated it should be discussed fully with the mother and her supporters in advance.

It will be difficult to determine with certainty whether the infant has been infected with HIV. Parents will face a prolonged period of uncertainty which may have an adverse effect on postnatal recovery and family adjustment. Preparation for transfer home should take account of these factors. The support available to her from the community midwife and health visitor should be emphasised, and arrangements for an initial paediatric follow up appointment should be confirmed. Education of parents to recognise and report significant signs of infection in the baby, linked with surveillance by the health visitor and/or GP is desirable.

The baby should be immunised in accordance with the routine schedule as recommended by the Joint Committee on Vaccination and Immunisation, except that BCG vaccine should be omitted (Joint Committee on Vaccination and Immunisation 1988).

■ Recommendations for clinical practice in the light of currently available evidence

A constructive response to HIV infection must include the following aspects.

1. Re-examination of, and improvement in standards of, clinical practice so that procedures confer minimal risk to clients and staff alike.

2. Measures of infection control that are neither threatening nor offensive to the women in our care.

3. A challenging of judgemental attitudes which interfere with women receiving tolerant and compassionate care.

4. Vigilant protection of the confidentiality of all women.

5. A commitment by midwives to keep themselves well informed.

Midwives are in a position to make a unique contribution to the care of women who are at risk of, or who have acquired, HIV infection. What we offer in terms of education, awareness and support will have an impact on the difficult future faced by these women and their babies. Our responsibility is to make that contribution a positive one.

■ Practice check

- Identify three areas in which midwives could develop their role as health educators/promotors in relation to HIV infection.

- List the clinical procedures which might put a midwife at risk of contamination by potentially infectious body fluids. What measures can you propose to eliminate these risks? How will you implement such measures in your place of work?

- You are looking after a woman who is HIV antibody positive. In what way do you think the confidentiality of the diagnosis might be jeopardised
    - antenatally?
    - in labour?
    - postnatally?
    - after transfer home?

- What strategies do you think need to be implemented to ensure that confidentiality is protected?

- What advice would you give to an HIV antibody positive woman at the time of discharge from midwifery care about monitoring the health of her baby?

■ References

Berrebi P J, Puel J, Tricoire J, Grandjean H, Herne P, Pontonnier G 1988 The influence of pregnancy on the evolution of the HIV infection. IV International Conference on AIDS Stockholm, June 1988; abstract 4041

Berthier A, Chamaret S, Fauchet R et al 1986 Transmissibility of human immunodeficiency virus in haemophiliac and non-haemophiliac children living in a private school in France. Lancet ii: 598–601

Biggar R J, Pahwa S, Minkoff H et al 1989 Immunosuppression in pregnant women infected with human immunodeficiency virus. American Journal of Obstetrics and Gynecology   161(5): 1239–44

Bradbeer C 1987 Is infection with HIV a risk factor for cervical intraepithelial neoplasia? Lancet   ii: 1277–78

Chin J 1988 The global patterns and prevalence of HIV infection in women. In Hudson C, Sharp F (eds) AIDS and obstetrics and gynaecology. Proceedings of the 19th Royal College of Obstetrics & Gynaecology Study Group. RCOG, London

Department of Health 1990 Guidance for health care workers: protection against infection with HIV and hepatitis viruses. HMSO, London

Gill N, Porter K 1989 Occupational transmission of HIV: summary of published reports. Unpublished paper. PHLS Communicable Disease Surveillance Centre, London

Henderson D J 1988 HIV infection: risks to health care workers and infection control. Nursing Clinics of North America   23: 767–77

Johnstone F D, MacCallum L, Brettle R, Inglis J M, Peutherer J F 1988 Does infection with HIV affect the outcome of pregnancy? British Medical Journal   296: 467

Joint Committee on Vaccination and Immunisation 1988 Immunisation against infectious disease. HMSO, London

Jovaisas E, Koch M A, Schafer A et al 1986 LAV/HTLVII virus in a 20 week fetus. Lancet   ii: 1129

MacCallum L R, France A J, Jones M E, Steel C M, Burns S M, Brettle R P et al 1988 The effects of pregnancy on the progression of HIV infection. IV International Conference on AIDS Stockholm, June 1988; abstract 4032

Miller D 1987 Counselling (ABC of AIDS). British Medical Journal   294: 167–74

Minchin M 1988 AIDS & breastmilk: the impact on women and babies. MIDIRS Information Pack, August

Minkoff H L 1987 Care of pregnant women infected with human immunodeficiency virus. Journal of the American Medical Association 285: 2714–17

Minkoff H L, Nanda D, Menez R, Fikrig S 1987 Pregnancies resulting in infants with AIDS or AIDS-related complex: follow-up of mothers, children, and subsequently born siblings. Obstetrics and Gynecology   69: 288–91

Mok J 1988 Infants of women seropositive for HIV. Midwife, Health Visitor and Community Nurse   24: 458–62

Mok J 1989 Babies of HIV infected women in Edinburgh. Midwifery   5: 17–20

Morbidity & Mortality Weekly Report 1987 Recommendations for prevention of HIV transmission in health-care settings. Report No 36, Supplement 2S: 3S–18S

Morbidity and Mortality Weekly Report 1988 Update: universal precautions for prevention of transmission of HIV, Hepatitis B virus and other bloodborne pathogens in health care settings. Report No 3: 24

New Scientist 1988 Fewer women agree to the test. 35

Nsa W, Ryder R W, Baende E, Kashamuka M, Francis H, Behets F, Davachi F 1988 Mortality from perinatally-acquired HIV infection in African children. IV International Conference on AIDS, June 1988; abstract 4126

Peckham C S, Senturia Y D, Ades A E, Newell M L 1988 Mother-to-child transmission of HIV infection: the European collaborative study. Lancet ii: 1039–42

Royal College of Nursing 1988 Nursing guidelines on the management of patients in hospital and the community suffering from AIDS. Second Report of the RCN AIDS working party. RCN, London

Rubinstein A, Bernstein L 1986 The epidemiology of pediatric AIDS. Clinical immunology and immunopathology 40: 115–21

Ryder R W, Hassig S 1988 The epidemiology of perinatal transmission of HIV. AIDS 2 (supplement 1): S83–89

Ryder R W, Nsa W, Behets F, Vercauteren G, Baende E, Lubaki M, Baudoux, Quinn T, Piot P 1988a Perinatal transmission in two African hospitals: one year follow-up. IV International Conference on AIDS, Stockholm, June 1988, abstract 4128

Ryder R W, Rayfield M, Quinn T C, Kashamuka M, Francis H, Vercauteren G, Piot P 1988b Transplacental transmission in African newborns. IV International Conference on AIDS, June 1988; abstract 5123

Schoenbaum E E, Davenny K, Selwyn P A 1988 The impact of pregnancy on HIV-related disease. In Hudson C, Sharp F (eds) AIDS and obstetrics and gynaecology. Proceedings of the 19th Royal College of Obstetrics and Gynaecology Study Group. RCOG, London

Schaefer A, Grosch-Woerner I, Friedmann W, Kunze R, Mielke M, Jimenez E 1988 The effects of pregnancy on the natural course of the HIV infection. IV International Conference on AIDS, June 1988l abstract 4039

Scott G B, Fischl M A, Klimas N et al 1985 Mothers of infants with the acquired immunodeficiency syndrome. Evidence for both symptomatic and asymptomatic carriers. Journal of the American Medical Association 253: 363–66

Scrimgeour J B 1988 Safety of invasive procedures in diagnostic antenatal and intrapartum care. In Hudson C, Sharp F (eds) AIDS and obstetrics and gynaecology. Proceedings of the 19th Royal College of Obstetrics and Gynaecology Study Group. RCOG, London

Semprini A E, Vucetich A, Pardi G et al 1986 HIV infection and AIDS in newborn babies of mothers positive for HIV antibody. British Medical Journal 294: 610

Sprecher S, Soumenkoff G, Puissant F et al 1986 Vertical transmission of HIV in a 15 week fetus. Lancet ii: 288–89

Thiry L, Sprecher-Goldberger, S, Jockheer T et al 1985 Isolation of AIDS virus from cell free breast milk of three healthy virus carriers. Lancet ii: 891–92

United Kingdom Central Council 1987 Circular PC/87/02. UKCC, London

Vogt M W, Witt D J, Craven D E et al 1986 Isolation of HTLVIII/LAV from cervical secretions of women at risk for AIDS. Lancet i: 525–27

Weiblen B J, Lee F K, Cooper E R, Landesman S H *et al* 1990 Early diagnosis of HIV infection in infants by detection of IgA HIV antibodies. Lancet i: 988–90
World Health Organisation 1987 Statement from the consultation on breast-feeding/breast milk and HIV. WHO, Geneva

■ Suggested further reading

Brierley J, Roth C 1989 Midwifery and AIDS – a users' guide. Nursing and AIDS series. Department of Health, London
Connor S, Kingman S 1988 The search for the virus. Penguin Books, Harmondsworth
Hudson C N, Sharp F (eds) 1988 AIDS in obstetrics and gynaecology. Proceedings of the 19th Study Group of the Royal College of Obstetricians and Gynaecologists. RCOG, London
Journal of Nurse-Midwifery 34(5): whole issue, September/October 1989
Richardson D 1989 Women and the AIDS crisis, 2nd ed. Pandora Press, London

Index

Note: numerals in **bold** type refer to volumes:
1 – Antenatal Care
2 – Intrapartum Care
3 – Postnatal Care